ford Poisoned
Himself, is Claim

ence Counsel Sees It as Only Answer to Man Staying in House.

DENCE IS ANALYZED

ements by Accused man's Husband Called Fantastic.

GOXXX, Oct. 1.—(CP)—A three.. address to the jury by C. W. K.C chief defence counsel, d the closing phases to-day of al of middle-aged Mrs. Elisa-Tilford for the poison murder of -year-old teamster husband.

Bell, physically unable to con-when Mr. Justice Kingstone ad-d the court until to-morrow g, declared that Tyrrel Til-had himself taken the arsenic which caused his death and d as "fantastic," statements by the deceased in the closing f his life.

court returns to-morrow Mr. ill continue his address and followed by Crown Attorney nyder. The defence did not pre-py witnesses and the crown ded its case before the noon nment after the 83rd witness en heard. It is expected the ill go to the jury to-morrow you imagine," Mr. Bell asked ry, "a man with a scrap of calmly lying in the house he believed he was being pois-of asking the doctor or his try rs to get him out)?

"Taking it himself."

at is the answer? There was found in his body—not to kill him, but it was there, is only one answer—that he ting it himself."

ell argued many remarks made sses had arisen from "fantas-ements" made by Tilford and the jurors to take no stock in which he said were involved case much more than in the s case.

Tilford, three times a widow d nervous as Mr. Bell made marks to the jury and often her face with a handkerchief. ising the evidence of some es, Mr. Bell stated that Mrs. ne Argent had said the accused dered arsenic and that her r was afraid to take it in. gave then failed to tell this inquest, which was strange if ry were true, he added. . ains woman had told another bout a note from Mrs. Tilford her not to get "mixed up" to as happening and concluding urn," Mr. Bell continued:-As such a note was written, suggested she would have Don't get me mixed up to." n't get mixed up in."

"Told it All."

good friend burned this note e was ever a note" and then it and told it all to at least wspaper reporter, and later and got him a photograph

Kingston General Hospital, where clinical work with ensol is proceeding.

Connell Assistant Not a College Man

Started Career in Laboratory Washing Out Test Tubes

ONLY 31 YEARS OLD

A laboratory assistant barely out of his twenties, who never had any university training and gained his first experience as a research worker by washing dishes, to-day shares with Dr. H. C. Connell of Kingston credit for the development of ensol and its preparation as a cancer treatment.

B. J. Holsgrove, Dr. Connell's bacteriological technician and chief assistant, is only 31 years old. Yet throughout the research which produced ensol, Dr. Connell depended (and still depends) upon Mr. Hols-grove for the actual performance of the important laboratory experiments, the details of the long process of trial and error with test tube and laboratory animals, and finally, the production of supplies of ensol itself for administration to cancer patients.

Mr. Holsgrove is little inclined to discuss this, but prefers to stress the point that the origin, nature and direction of the entire research emanated from Dr Connell, that the long labor for success was conduct-ed throughout under the close sur-

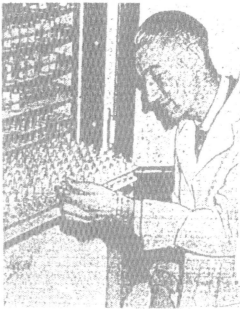

B. J. Holsgrove, laboratory technician, inspecting refrigerator tray tiny bottles containing ensol.

Discoverer of Ensol
Only 40 Years O

It is from this particular field,
namely the study of the serological processes
involved in immunity and disease,
that, success in treatment and control of cancer
will be found.

HENDRY C. CONNELL, 1895-1964

[C]ancer Relief Claimed Fo[r]

[Ne]wly-Discovered 'Ensol' [Di]ssolves Cancer Growth [--] Kingston Medico Reports

NEW CANCER TREATM[ENT]

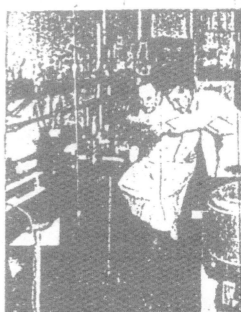

[Rese]arches on 30 Pa[tien]ts Show Benefits of [Tre]atment — Experi[men]ts Continue

Returns $39,000 Dime Is Reward

Youth Finds Fortune and Gets Little

[Se]ptember, 1935, Dr. Hendry [Connel]l, of Queen's University, [wh]o commenced his researches [which] have led to his new treat[ment for] cancer.

In the current issue of the [Canadia]n Medical Association Jour[nal he] is able to report the results [of] treatment on 30 cases "which [we]nt home to die."

[Of th]ese 30 cases, four did die [the] remaining 26 some of them [seem] to be completely relieved o[f pa]in and have definitely im[proved], others have slight relief [but] pain has been relieved but [gene]ral condition has not im[proved].

[The] cases seem to respond after [a few] days' treatment," Dr. Con[nell repo]rts. "In the group of cases [at prese]nt under observation the ef[fects a]re consistently good. There [is] a marked gain in weight, [disa]ppearance of severe cach[exia] (Cachexia—faulty nutrition) [the] growths have shown arrest, [soft]ening and absorption. In [case]s where pain has been a [consta]nt symptom the sedatives [have be]en cut in half and in many [cases di]scontinued.

[V]ACCINE TREATMENT

[Th]e internal growths a similar [... is] apparently going on [a] great deal of clinical im[proveme]nt has been noted."

[The] treatment consists of intra[muscular] or intravenous injections [of a] solution developed by Dr.

The treatment, generally [speaking], is based on the theory that [seru]m, or vaccine, from a body [that h]as been inoculated with the [... di]sease has the power to [treat that] disease in another body, [se]rum and vaccine used against [diphther]ia and smallpox, respective [... ex]amples. Ensol, however, is [neither] a serum nor a vaccine. It [is a sol]ution prepared from cancer [it]self.

[...] cases have been treated [...] purely from the clinical [point of] view. Detailed biochemical [reac]tions of the body fluids are [un]dertaken. Cytological (cy[tology—]the science of cell-formation [and ...]life) studies of the cancer [com]paring biopsy specimens be[fore and] after treatment are being [...]

St. Louis, Oct. 2—For returning a [$3]9,000 bank cheque he had found [Wo]ody Robinson, 16-year-old mes[s]enger boy, received a dime reward [y]esterday.

As the youth was crossing the [st]reet he noticed a slip of paper cov[er]ed with blue marks. Picking it up, [h]e saw it was a Mississippi Valley [T]rust Company cheque for $39,000 [en]dorsed "David E. Woods, 12 Garns[w]ald Park."

Woody took it to the bank and an [a]ttendant summoned the man who [h]ad been carrying the cheque to the [ba]nk to deposit it.

"The man seemed awfully happy," [W]oody said. "He dug down in his [p]ocket and pulled out a nickel, then [t]old me he thought it was worth [m]ore than that and handed me a [di]me."

Woody declined to comment fur[th]er.

[the] tumor cells in various degrees [o]f destruction.

"During the progress of the ani[m]al experiments several cases of [C]arcinoma were under my care with [t]he condition. They had been pro[n]ounced incurable and sent home to [d]ie, after all forms of recognized [m]odern treatment had been applied. [The]se were given human carcinoma [E]nsol intramuscularly. There was [no] inflammatory or other systemic [re]action .... The immediate results [we]re most remarkable and quite un[l]ike anything previously observed.

"To verify and confirm these results [I] naturally sought other cases which [c]ould only be secured by announcing [the] discovery to my colleagues and [so]liciting their cooperation and as[s]istance. This has been most gener[ou]sly rendered. As are would ex[pe]ct, the type of cases which we felt [j]ustified in treating were only those [c]onsidered hopeless from the point [o]f view of all recognized forms of [t]reatment. In spite of this severe [te]st the treatment has produced re[su]lts which, we feel confirm our [ea]rlier observations.

HORSE SERUM

Writing from the clinical standpoint, [D]r. Connell states: "When the first

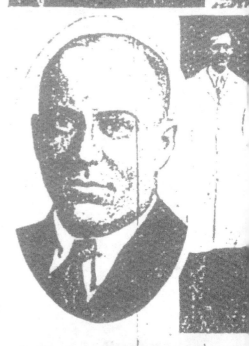

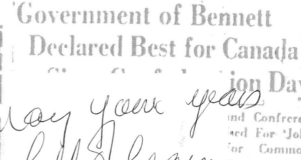

gston Doctor's Treatment

OPED AT KINGSTON

'Government of Bennett Declared Best for Canada

May your years be full of learning & thrills to Love

on Day

nd Confere ed For 'Jol or Commo

Must Not Have Been In Vain

Robert &
Katherine Connell Crothers

Nana + Bippa

Ex-Calgarian Asks Divorce

General A. C. Critchley, British M.P., Cites Orchestra Leader

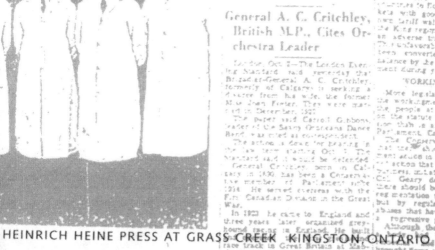

HEINRICH HEINE PRESS AT GRASS CREEK KINGSTON ONTARIO

BookSurge, LLC
www.booksurge.com
1-866-308-6235
orders@booksurge.com

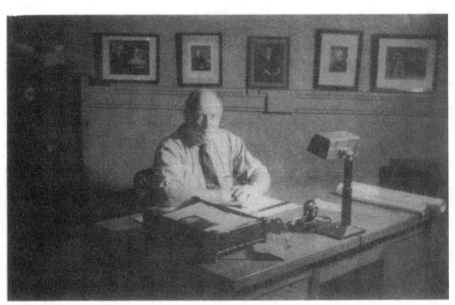

H.C. Connell, February 1947

PREFACE

I saw my father cry only once. It was on Wednesday morning, March 30, 1938.

He sat with his head in his hands at the breakfast table, his cheeks wet with tears. The usual family discussion about the radio news of the day with my uncle Ken wasn't taking place. I couldn't believe that my wonderful father, who wiped other people's tears and solved their problems, including mine, was crying.

My heart sank. The reason for my father's tears came soon enough. He had learned from one of his medical colleagues in Florida that some of their patients had died during cancer treatment in Orlando. They had been given a contaminated injection of a serum that my father had developed.

At home, with his family around him, the physician and researcher, could show his true feelings.

This book is about my father, Calvin Hendry Cameron Connell, a Canadian living in Kingston,Ontario. He was a physician and medical researcher whose pioneering work, successes and struggles led to early treatments for cancer. He developed an enzyme solution he named Ensol, which proved to dissolve cancer cells.

No cure for cancer has yet been found. But Ensol, and all the other treatments that have followed it, bettered the lives of cancer patients. Research has come a long way since my father's work, but it doesn't seem fast enough for most of us.

We hope this story of Hendry Connell and Ensol will interest all those whose lives have been touched by cancer, whether they are patients, their family, friends or acquaintances.

Kingston was the site of the development and discovery of Ensol. By the late fall of 1935, Queen's University and the Kingston hospitals were assisting in the necessary clinical work.

This is a story that should have been told long ago, but wasn't. It begins on the following pages with the announcement of the discovery of Ensol in the *Queen's Review* of August 1935.

KATHERINE CROTHERS

ACKNOWLEDGEMENTS

For their dedication and faith in Hendry's cause and for their assistance in our research, we want to thank three supportive employees of the Hendry-Connell Research Foundation: Donald K. Alexander, (chemist), now living in Wellington, Ontario; Anne Preston Caldwell, (secretary), Kingston, Ontario; and Dr. Ralph Glasser, (bacteriologist), Tuscon, Arizona.

To Dr. Wendell Shackelford we are most indebted. He kept us on an even keel and on course. His optimism is contagious.

Amongst many others who contributed to this story, we are also grateful to Marcia Weese of the Queen's University Archives; the *Orlando Sentinel* Archive researchers; the Philadelphia Free Library; health records analyst Shelly Broome, Hotel Dieu Hospital, Kingston; Gary Rivers for his skill and patience in copying; Dr. Bev Lynn for his biography of Dr. J.C.; and Peter Dorn for his cover and book design, and for his editorial help. We are also grateful for their advice to Steve Lukits, *The Kingston Whig-Standard;* and to Joan Harcourt. The late Professor Frederick Gibson's volume on the history of Queen's University was very helpful to us.

Finally, our thanks to our children – Katherine, Robert, Gordon and Sandy – for their interest in the project and for their skills.

 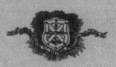

The QUEEN'S REVIEW

Official Publication of the General Alumni Association
of Queen's University.

Vol. 9   KINGSTON, ONT., AUGUST, 1935   No. 6

TABLE OF CONTENTS

The QUEEN'S REVIEW is published monthly, October to May inclusive, and in August. Annual subscription is $3.00. If subscriber is an alumnus of Queen's, REVIEW subscription is included in the annual membership dues of the General Alumni Association.

Editor and Business Manager—Gordon J. Smith, B.A., B.Sc.

Assistant Editors—J. Lorne MacDougall, B.A.
            Anna F. Corrigan, B.A.

Address all communications to the QUEEN'S REVIEW, General Alumni Association, Douglas Library, Queen's University, Kingston.

PRINTED AND BOUND BY THE JACKSON PRESS, KINGSTON, ONT

CHAPTER 1

THE DISCOVERY OF ENSOL

reprinted from
The Queen's Review, August 1935, Vol 9, No 6, page 169

The discovery of a treatment that, in the guarded phraseology of an earlier formal pronouncement, is apparently capable of arresting the development of cancer and may lead to its ultimate control, earns for Dr. Hendry C. Connell, and incidentally for Queen's University and Canada, the plaudits of the scientific world. The *Review* adds its very sincere congratulations to those being showered upon Dr. Connell by the alumni of Queen's and the medical profession.

A cautious preliminary statement revealing the general lines of his research and the results obtained was released by Dr. Connell during July. In this announcement Dr. Connell stated that he had developed an entirely new series of biological products – which he had named "Ensols"– one of which was apparently capable of arresting the growth of carcinoma cancer and might control it. The statement was given out reluctantly, as it was regarded as premature, but it was deemed necessary on account of wide-spread rumours concerning the patients under treatment and other phases of the work being done.

That this splendid contribution should have been made here will afford Queen's men and women reason for pride. It is very gratifying to think that if Dr. Connell's work bears out the high promise it holds at present it will give Queen's a noted and enviable place among the world's scientific institutions. Even if the Ensol treatment should not prove a complete success in controlling cancer, it has opened up a new field of hope and endeavour. In the words of the Toronto *Globe*, "If his early hopes and results are in any way borne out by further tests,

Dr. Connell should have placed at his disposal at least some reasonable proportion of the King's Jubilee Cancer Fund, now stated to have reached a total of $437,000 ... If by his work Dr. Connell has achieved something that will even point the way to a cure and assist others in going further, he is entitled to unstinted acclaim." In this sentiment the *Review* heartily concurs. With cancer clinics already established in connection with the University and the Kingston hospitals, and with cancer work of such paramount importance going on here, Queen's might well be chosen as the site of a cancer institute. Those with money at their disposal for cancer research should give serious consideration to the wisdom of building on what Dr. Connell, with his industry and resourcefulness has accomplished.

Adding not a little to the credit due Dr. Connell for his discovery is the fact that his research was carried on almost single-handed and in the face of many obstacles. Not the least of his difficulties was the lack of adequate financial assistance and of laboratory facilities. A grant of $500 was secured from the National Research Council for services and supplies when the biological problem of cataract was under investigation, but aside from that the expense of the research has been borne by Dr. Connell himself. The cost of the work so far has run into thousands of dollars.

No final claims have been put forward as yet by Dr. Connell regarding his achievement. Only a very careful statement of facts has come from the laboratories where he and his valued assistant have been working for four years. But that cautious statement reveals a discovery that may prove the greatest advance in the whole study of cancer. Time is, of course, the test upon which the scientific world will insist; but medical men have already said that the facts disclosed indicate a remarkable discovery.

Associated with Dr. Connell in the work and deserving of much praise is Bertram Holsgrove, a technician in the Bacteriology department. Mr. Holsgrove furnished a great deal of the expert technical background needed in the experimentation of the laboratory work. No small amount of credit must also be given to two men who were Dr. Connell's mainstays in the way of support, advice and encouragement. They are his father, Dr. J.C. Connell, the former Dean of Medicine, and Dr. A.L. Clark, Chairman of the University's Committee on Scientific Research.

Dr. Connell feels that there is no doubt about the fundamental nature of his discovery and is now testing it fully by applying it to all sorts of cancer cases. If what has already been repeatedly demonstrated continues to be verified by more general use – if it is established that a blood-carried biochemical product destroys cancer cells and their products but is harmless to the normal organism – the benefits to the human race will be beyond computation.

End of *The Queen's Review*, August 1935, Vol 9, No 6, page 169.

The tone and the excitement apparent in the above article makes one wonder how such skill, energy and tenacity developed and were nurtured. Some answers lie in Hendry Cameron Connell's early years.

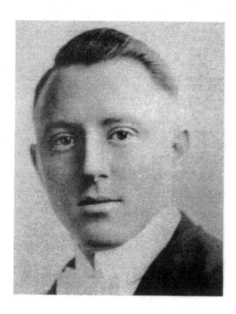

Hendry C. Connell
"Keeps his council, does his duty,
cleaves to friends
and loveth beauty."
*Year Book 1918, page 65,
Science – Arts – Medicine 1918*

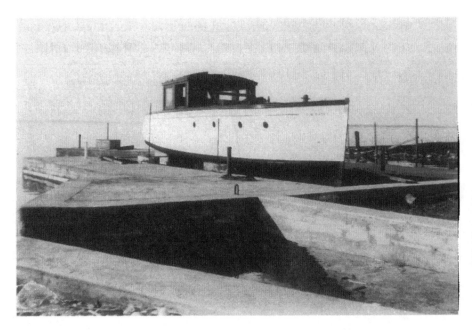

The *Jim-Katha*

CHAPTER 2

Calvin Hendry Cameron Connell was born in Kingston August 28th, 1895, the only son of Dr. J.C. Connell (Arts 1884, Meds.'88, LLD.) and his wife Agnes Hendry Connell.

What better time to be born. The closing years of the nineteenth century not only offered all the rapid changes and improvements in lifestyle and travel accomplished during the Victorian era of that century, but also held a bright image of newer and better things to be accomplished in the twentieth century. He became very familiar with jet-powered air travel during his lifetime.

As an infant Hendry developed a calcium deficiency disease which required his being carried on a pillow in his infancy. Living on King Street bordering the harbour, his interest in water and boats was readily stimulated. Young Connell was at home on the water and was an accomplished boatman at an early age. His first experience was with a small skiff fitted with a one-cylinder St. Lawrence gasoline engine: with exposed flywheel, spark plug, battery and brass priming cup. It was very easy to understand how these engines operated because everything was visible from the outside. By the late 1920's this same boatman built a 42-foot power cruiser powered by an eight-cylinder engine specifically designed for marine use.

His mother's grandfather was D.D. Calvin, founder of the Calvin Shipbuilding and Rafting Company of Garden Island. Hendry made the trip from Garden Island to Quebec City on the last raft this company sent down the 350 miles of St. Lawrence River for transhipment overseas. D.D. Calvin had sent his first raft on the same journey some ninety years before. This was a very successful local business begun early in the nineteenth century and whose history and accomplishments were actively experienced by Hendry Connell. What an oppor-

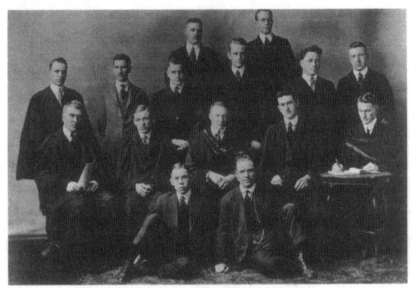

CONCURSUS INQUITATIS ET VIRTUTIS   SESSION '16 –'17
Row 1: F.B.Goodfellow, *Constable*; F.B. Sharp, *Jury*
Row 2: J.H. Scott, *Pros. Attorney*; J. Murphy, *Crier*; R.E. Page, Sheriff; C.M. Carruthers, *Constable*; C.W. Ferrell, *Constable*; D.R. Hall, *Constable*
Row 3: S.J.W. Horn, *Pros.Attorney*; L.C. Purvis, *Sr. Judge*; H.C.Connell, BA, *Chief Justice*
Row 4: C.H.McCuaig, *Jury*; B.D.Hunt, *Chief Constable*

tunity to start life with a good knowledge of the past and to take part in the future as it unfolded!

Hendry was educated at Kingston Victoria School and Kingston Collegiate Institute. He entered the Art's faculty at Queen's and received his BA in 1915. He then joined the class of Medicine '19 but secured his MD CM a year earlier due to the acceleration of classes during the war. Hendry was known as "Spec" in his college years because of his short stature. Prominent in athletics, he played interyear and interfaculty rugby and hockey. In second year Medicine, he was a member of the senior football team. A broken leg cut short his rugby career, however. In executive work he was a member of the Athletic Board, was president of Med. '19 in his third year and chief justice of the Concursus Iniquitatis et Virtutis of the Aesculapian Society.

At the end of the war he served as a medical officer in a Canadian Hospital at Vladivostok, Russia, where typhus fever was very prevalent. He then went on to further studies in London and Vienna before returning again to Kingston to enter practice with his father, and gradually to take over this extensive practice as a specialist in diseases of the eye, ear, nose and throat.

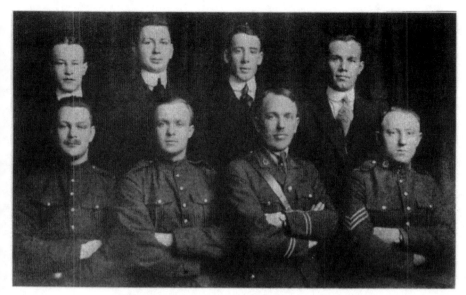

EXECUTIVE MEDICINE '19, THIRD (Summer) SESSION, 1916
D.L. MacDonell, *Historian*; E.M. McCoy, *Orator*; V.C. McCuaig, *Sec.-Treas*; F.B. Sharp, *Poet*
J.T. Fowkes, *Prophet*; J.R. Simmons, *Vice-Pres*; Dr. J.F. Sparks, *Hon. Pres*; H.C. Connell, *Pres.*

Hendry married Katie Reid of Kingston, daughter of Mr. and Mrs. Robert J. Reid on June 5th, 1918. They had three children: James Cameron (January 12th, 1920); Mary Katherine (March 8th, 1923); and Hendry Reid (December 24th, 1938).

In 1929 Hendry was appointed assistant professor in the faculty of medicine teaching the treatment of diseases in his specialties. By 1930 he had begun research in a laboratory set up on the third floor of the Queen's medical building to find a method of dissolving the cataract of the eye. It was private research, conducted on a part time basis and carried out after hours; his only assistant was a young laboratory technician, Bertram Holsgrove, who was associated with the department of Bacteriology at that time. The only money Hendry was granted was $500 by the National Research Council for his cataract research. Otherwise, he financed this research from his own funds.

He sought a product that would break down lens protein into soluble substances. He eventually found that by growing non-pathogenic proteolyic micro-organisms on protein media, which themselves liquefied in the process, an active substance or enzyme was produced. This could be separated from the other constituents of the media and made sterile, and was found to have the power of liquefying protein similar to its base while having no effect on other types. Dr. Connell demonstrated the specific character of this substance, showing that it would break down cataractous lens tissue without having any reaction on other proteins. He named it Ensol, from "enzyme" and "solution."

The positive laboratory results in connection with cataract research led Dr. Connell to visualize the application of this same principle to other diseases, especially the various forms of cancer. He directed his research to the production of an Ensol from a carcinoma base that might have a specific action upon carcinoma tissue. Mice infected with carcinoma were used to develop mouse Ensol and to demonstrate its action. Profound changes were produced in the tumor mass in mice within a few days of the initial treatment, and case histories of these tests were carefully kept, furnishing an indication of what might be expected to occur in the human body.

In early spring of 1935 came the use of Ensol upon carcinoma patients who had been pronounced incurable and inoperable by the most competent of medical men. No inflammatory action took place, and there was remarkable and immediate improvement in the general condition of each of the patients. Apparently the growth of the carcinoma was

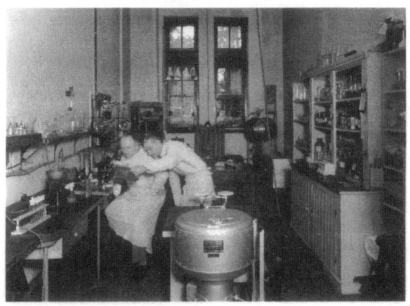

H.C. Connell and Bert Holsgrove in laboratory
Ontario Hall, Queen's University, 1935

arrested and the process reversed to one of retrogression. All the clinical results were uniform and amazing!

By 1935 Queen's had provided a better area for research in Ontario Hall where a room was placed at Connell's disposal. The university provided the quarters together with heat and power. Bars were installed on the windows for security as the research became newsworthy and grew in magnitude. Dr. Connell fitted out the laboratory at his own expense and carried the work forward. As he was carrying on his regular medical practice he could devote only the time after hours to the research. Together he and Bert Holsgrove laboured almost incessantly, utilizing Sundays, holidays and often most every night as they pressed on toward their goal. At this point Mr. Holsgrove's services were largely gratuitous.

The following article appeared in *The Kingston Whig-Standard,* Wednesday, July 17, 1935.

Discovery of Cancer Treatment Is Made at Queen's
Kingston Medical Research Worker Discovers Solution That Is Arresting Cancer

Dr. Hendry C. Connell Makes Announcement of World-wide Interest – Research Occupies Four Years – Patients Innoculated Here Show Distinct Improvement in Condition.

CARRIES DEATH TO CANCER CELLS

Great Advance in Treatment of Cancer - Solution Harmless to Normal Organism - Hoped That the Connell Ensol May Result in Checking Disease and Possibly Curing It.

From his laboratory at Queen's University, Kingston, Dr. Hendry C. Connell announces that he has discovered an entirely new series of biological products which he calls "Ensol," one of which arrests the development of carcinoma cancer and may control it. The solution is injected into the blood stream of the patient and therefore reaches every portion of the body.

In the summer of 1935 the *Canadian Medical Association Journal* published the preliminary report by Dr. Hendry C. Connell titled *The Study and Treatment of Cancer by proteolytic enzymes.* This was the first official pronouncement of the five years of research.

The press release, together with editorial comment by the *Journal* to the Canadian Press resulted in immediate awareness throughout North America of the extent and preliminary success of this research since 1930.

The following article appeared in *The Mail and Empire*, no longer published under this title, in July 1935.

Five Years' Research Produces New Weapon For Attack on Cancer

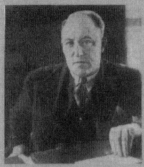

DR. H.C. CONNELL

Test Injections of Ensol in Human Bodies Appear To Ameliorate Disease, Kingston Doctor Reports – Warns Against Unjustifiable Hopes

Research by a Kingston physician has evolved a new treatment for cancer which may prove to be the means long sought by science to combat that disease.

The treatment involves injection of "Ensol," the name bestowed on the anti-cancer element discovered by Dr. H.C. Connell, originator and director of the research. In the several hundred cases thus far treated, retrogression of the cancerous growths has been achieved without discomfort or harmful effects accompanying the process in any case.

Correlated with the discovery of the new element is the revelation in a new light of a basic bio-chemical principle. Out of further application of this principle, it is hoped, may come not only abatement of the scourge of cancer, but discovery of similar elements for the combating of tuberculosis and other diseases for which specific curative elements are unknown.

Only Time Will Tell

Dr. Connell, who relinquished practice as an eye-ear-nose-throat specialist to devote all his time to the research, reflects the age-old caution of his profession. He is insistent that the element he has discovered, and produced for successful administration to humans, must not be described as a cancer cure.

Only time, patience and further tests lasting months or years will show definitely and conclusively, he avers, whether his discovery is what it now appears to be – an agent for both the eradication of cancerous growths and possible immunization against their development.

Nevertheless, with publication today in the **Journal of the Canadian Medical Association** of the first report of his research, every indication is that he has gone far along the road toward this goal. At least to the lay mind, medicine seems to have within reach, if not within its grasp, the means of achieving dissolution of the deadly growths in cancer sufferers.

Bio-chemical Principle

Great and hopeful as is the importance attached to Dr. Connell's anti-cancer agent, his projection of the bio-chemical principle on which it is based is felt to possess, at least potentially, even more significance. The principle is the simple, but hitherto neglected one, of tissue-consuming ferments, and already it is guiding extended research to determine its application to other diseases, tuberculosis in particular.

Those who have studied Dr. Connell's work and its results foresee, quite apart from the eventual value or otherwise of the new cancer treatment, that the basic principle involved will open a new field of medico-scientific investigation. Just as the discovery of insulin led the way to vast new knowledge in regard to bodily metabolism and the glands of internal secretion, so, it is believed, will Ensol result in vastly increased understanding of the chemistry and cellular structure of diseased body tissue.

Granted that further tests will confirm the ability of Ensol to dissolve cancerous tissues and diminish growths, the question to which medical science patiently and cautiously awaits the answer is this: Can Ensol check malignancy without injuring normal body tissues? Should the existing indications to this effect be confirmed by further and conclusive research, theories hitherto held as to the workings of tissue-destroying elements will be revolutionized.

This, of course, remains to be seen, but the record of Ensol's achievements thus far is clouded with no such element of conjecture. Patients' charts in the Kingston General Hospital, X-Ray plates made after Ensol treatments, confirm the visual evidence of patients who entered the hospital bed-ridden, racked by pain, but walked out unassisted to return to normal daily activities.

The following are comments made in publications across Canada after the announcement of the discovery of Ensol by Dr. Hendry Connell on the same date and the fall of 1935.

TORONTO, July 17 (CP) "Biochemistry may ultimately be an important factor in the solution of the cancer problem." Dr. W.J. Bell, Ontario deputy minister of health, said today when questioned concerning the discovery, announced by Dr. Hendry C. Connell of Kingston, of a new series of biological products he calls 'Ensols,' one of which has arrested development of carcinoma cancer and may control it.

Dr. Bell made the statement after carefully reading the description of Dr. Connell's discovery. He would offer no further comment.

Hon. J.A. Faulkner, minister of health, was out of the city.

"GOOD NEWS"

STELLARTON, N.S., July 17 (CP) "Good news, of course," said Dr. R.M. Benvie of Stellarton, president of the Nova Scotia Medical Society, when told of Dr. Hendry C. Connell's announced discovery at Kingston of new growths which may offer a cancer cure.

"But the stand of the medical profession in cases of this 'kind,' the doctor emphasized, "is that it must be shown. Very often, it has been found, good results will be obtained by one man, although his method will not work successfully in general use."

"But it's very good news," the doctor repeated: "And coming from a responsible authority, will carry considerable weight. Doubtless this announcement would not have been made unless there was a solid basis for it."

American Opinion

NEW YORK, July 17 (CP) "Bitter experience has taught us to accept all announcements of discoveries on the cause and cure of cancer with the utmost caution," Dr. Iago Galdston, executive secretary of the information bureau of the New York Academy of Medicine, said today on being informed of the reported discovery of a possible cancer control by Dr. Hendry Connell.

"In this instance we have not even the benefit of the research protocols, since, according to Dr. Connell's announcement, the detailed reports of his work are yet to be published in a scientific journal.

The press release is of the vaguest character as far as scientific particulars are concerned. Hence, there is no basis upon which even presumptively one might opine on the work.

"The claims made by Dr. Connell are most extraordinary. At the present and until such time as dependable proof is forthcoming, all we can say is that the announcement is most remarkable, if correct."

Medical Journal Endorses Work Of Kingston Man

Editorial Bespeaks Aid for Doctor in Cancer Research

WAITS DEVELOPMENTS

Results so Far Justify Continuance, Official Organ Declares

Discovery by Dr. H. C. Connell of Kingston of a new treatment for cancer and his continuing research into its value, are the subject of congratulatory editorial comment in the October issue of the Canadian Medical Association Journal,published today. The comment is initialed by Dr. A.G. Nicholls, editor of the Journal.

After noting that "much interest has been aroused both in lay and medical circles" by the treatment, the lengthy editorial draws "particular attention" to a preliminary report by Dr. Connell appearing in the same issue of the Journal.

The editorial says further, in part, "So many cancer 'cures' are being reported these days that the medical profession at large has developed an attitude of horrid incredulity in regard to them, to the extent that it is almost impossible for the research worker who has a new idea to bring it forward with any hope of having it judged on its merits. We are glad to know that Dr. Connell is in a more favorable position. He has associated with him a number of men of high repute in the profession, representing various aspects of medicine, men capable of weighing evidence.

Thoroughly Scientific

"We are sure his work is being thoroughly and scientifically carried on, and that his conclusions, whatever they may eventually prove to be, will be accepted as accurate. Those who have seen the cases of cancer under his treatment have been impressed with the results he can show, which, to say the least, are encouraging. Certainly, his work cannot be lightly passed by..."

Doctors Cautious On Connell Find

Toronto physicians last night described Dr. H.C. Connell's Ensol discoveries as exceedingly interesting, but declined further comment at the present stage. It would be at least a year before anything approaching a conclusive verdict could be given, they said. As soon as Ensol is available it will be tried out clinically here, a member of the faculty of medicine said.

Dr.Connell Praised By St.Thomas Man
F.B. Holtby Took "Ensol" Treatment in Kingston Hospital

ST.THOMAS, Oct. 3 Praise for Dr. Hendry C. Connell of Kingston and serum he is using in the treatment of cancer was offered yesterday by F.B. Holtby of this city, former local bank manager. Mr. Holtby has returned after spending six weeks at Kingston and undergoing treatment.

"I was among the first to go to Kingston and became well acquainted with Dr. Connell," Mr. Holtby said. "Before I left over 200 persons were receiving the Ensol. I made it my duty to talk to all the men there for treatment, and I did not meet a case which had not benefited in a marvelous degree. They were there from all over Canada and the United States and many of the cases were very far advanced. It appeared to me that miracles were being performed."

Fifteen Patients Are Being Treated at the Hotel Dieu Clinic

The cancer clinic at the Hotel Dieu Hospital, which opened over two weeks ago, has been an extremely busy part of the hospital. Patients have been receiving treatment at the Hotel Dieu clinic, some leaving and returning later for further treatment. At the present time there are fifteen patients receiving treatment at the cancer clinic at the Hotel Dieu.

Patients from distant points comprise the list of patients receiving treatment at the clinic. Visits are made to the hospital regularly by doctors administering the Ensol treatment. Several cases have been reported as being materially helped by the treatment although, it was pointed out, no cures are claimed.

Further Comments Cancer Discovery Of Dr. H.C. Connell

VANCOUVER, July 10 (CP) "It is a credit to the work being done in Canadian cancer research centers," stated Dr. Wesley C. Prowd, in charge of cancer treatments at St. Paul's Hospital, Vancouver, commenting on 'Ensol' as announced by Dr. Hendry C. Connell of Queen's University, Kingston.

"A good deal of research has been done to try to discover a cure of this nature," Dr. Prowd said. "The theory is there may be a serum or solution that may be used against cancer in much the same way certain serums are used against typhoid and smallpox."

Montreal View

MONTREAL, July 10 (CP) Commenting on the announcement by Dr. H.C. Connell of Queen's University, Kingston, Ont., of a carcinoma cure for cancer, Dr. Edward Archibald of Royal Victoria Hospital, noted Montreal cancer specialist, said:

"Every fresh 'discovery' concerning the cause or cure of cancer demands careful consideration and investigation by those of the medical profession who have any competency of judgment.

"One note of caution which must be heard is: 'Foreign protein injected into the blood of cancer patients has sometimes produced extraordinary immediate improvement with ultimately curing the disease,'" he declared. "Intercurrent bacterial injections have done the same."

Approving Editorial

Over the signature of A.G. Nicholls, its editor, the same issue of the Medical Association Journal carries a restrained and carefully worded editorial, which, nevertheless, constitutes a congratulation of Dr. Connell.

The editorial states that the new treatment has "distinct promise," and expresses full confidence in the sincerity and motives of Dr. Connell and his associates. "The degree of amelioration which he has obtained is distinctly encouraging, and clearly demands that his work be continued," it adds.

During the summer and fall of 1935, many North American newspapers continued to print news stories of the development of Ensol and of the promising results experienced by those doctors administering it to their patients. These stories ensured the broadest circulation to a fascinated public. This sudden and somewhat unexpected volume of publicity was of considerable concern to Hendry, and was the subject of a letter from him to another colleague referring to an article in the December 14th 1935 issue of *Liberty* magazine. In his letter Hendry indicated that the article was responsible not only for an exceptional increase in letters of inquiry but also an increase of patients arriving on the doorstep requesting treatment. These developments put additional stress on the whole operation. A newspaper story at the time indicated that the influx of patients was tending to make it difficult for Queen's students to find room and board in the neighborhood as readily as in previous years.

Although *Liberty* magazine is no longer published, it was a weekly magazine with wide circulation in the US and Canada. Each item or article was always given a reading time and this article by a staff writer named Edward Doherty was labeled 8 minutes, 5 seconds. This article was certainly presented as sensational despite the Editor's Note: "Dr. Connell asks *Liberty* to make it very plain that his facilities are limited and no patients can be treated who are not recommended by their own physicians after consultation and correspondence with his office. In publishing this article, *Liberty*, of course is not endorsing Dr. Connell's remedy." The editor, Bernard Macfadden, commented; "Of course *Liberty* presents this article because of its news interest."

Dr. Connell had not provided any Ensol to doctors outside Kingston before July 1935, with the exception of one shipment. Following the publication of his research, a radio telephone call which traversed nearly twenty thousand miles of space, from Dr. Neville Davis in Sydney, Australia, urgently requested a supply of Ensol for a cancer patient. A supply, carefully refrigerated, was sent to Toronto by motor and from there flown to San Francisco and placed on board a liner, the *SS Mariposa*. On the ship's approach to Australia it was met by an aeroplane and the shipment transferred and flown on to Sydney. There is no record of the elapsed time for the whole trip, but the doctor there treated three patients and requested a further supply. Dr. Davis was to become a keen contributor to the clinical development of Ensol.

There was a report in a Toronto newspaper dated 1st October telling of a man convicted of a bank robbery who was just beginning to serve his term at Kingston Penitentiary when stricken with stomach cancer. Given up by doctors and surgeons, he was transferred to the Kingston General Hospital on the verge of death. It was there Dr. Connell saw him and began treatment with Ensol. As continued in the newspaper story,

> Officialdom at Ottawa, convinced that the grimmest scourge of nature had taken the case out of their hands, put through a pardon. The felon would at least die a free man. But he didn't die and he isn't dead. And, although Dr. Connell's associates vigorously and emphatically refuse to say that he has made a full recovery, the man now has a good appetite, good colour and has gained thirty-two pounds. Only a few days ago he telephoned a cheery goodbye to Dr. Connell before setting off to visit relatives in the Maritimes.

By the end of 1935, the administration required to organize and staff clinics was being enthusiastically assembled by skilled doctors who had already had experience with Ensol and were prepared to assume responsibility as department heads. Both Kingston hospitals, the General and the Hotel Dieu, were being used for Connell cancer clinics.

Dr. Connell insisted that the discovery was not to be exploited or any charge to be made. It was to be used wholly for those afflicted with cancer.

CHAPTER 3

From Frederick W. Gibson's Queen's University History, Volume II, 1917-1961 entitled *to serve and yet be free* as well as the minutes of the Board of Trustees and its executive committee, we learn of the whirlwind that surrounded Hendry Connell in the last six months of the year 1935. Professor Gibson's detailed descriptions of these ongoing events tell how the development of the Hendry-Connell Research Foundation came about so quickly and the pressures that were generated from all sides to accomplish the close association with the university if only for the three year period agreed on.

By the year 1935 Dr. Hendry Connell had relinquished his practice, devoting all his time to the research and financing all costs from his own resources. He continued to seek further additional funds from other sources as well as from Queen's University.

Hendry attended, by invitation, a meeting of the executive committee of the Board of Trustees on July 23rd, 1935 and gave a report on his laboratory and clinical work in the field of cancer research. As a result of this meeting, a committee was formed to discuss financial assistance with representatives of the Faculty of Medicine and hospital authorities.

Minutes of a meeting called by the Dean of the Medical Faculty, Dr. Frederic Etherington, held on 25th July, 1935, report the following resolutions passed:

1. The research at present being carried out on cancer by Dr. Hendry Connell is worthy of support from the University.
2. Prolonged investigation is necessary in order to establish the real worth of claims put forward.
3. Cooperation to be maintained with a committee of the Medical Faculty.
4. Association of the clinical aspects of Connell's researches with the cancer clinic which had been set up at the Kingston General Hospital in 1933 with the aid of the Provincial Government.

15

Cooperation by the hospital included adding to the hospital employment list Connell's laboratory staff for specific purposes, as well as the provision of an office for filing progress records. In return, Dr. Connell was to add to his clinic as consultants, professors from the medicine and surgery departments. On this foundation, the executive committee agreed to commend to the trustees at their upcoming fall meeting that $4,000 be granted to Hendry Connell for equipment and supply requirements for use in the university space presently occupied.

Before this expected fall meeting of the Board of Trustees took place when the executive committees' report would be received and presumably acted upon, a number of developments were in motion or had taken place. There were some, including Principal Fyfe, who felt that too close a connection between the university and the Connell research on cancer could easily subject the Board of Trustees to censure. The principal, in a note to the chairman of the Board, J.M. Macdonnell, indicated that he did not want the university completely separate from the Connell research, but neither to commit itself to co-operating.

The principal's inclination to remain non-committal appears to have coincided with Dr. Connell's intentions at this time. He had requested that the matter of assistance by Queen's be delayed.

However, at the fall Board of Trustees meeting held on Saturday, 12th October 1935, there were many members of the board who indicated that a "further effort" should be made to establish a close connection with the now existing Hendry-Connell Research Foundation. The apparent urgency taken after agreement on Miss Whitton's motion would indicate such a desire by the board.

Further developments are best told from the minutes of the Board of Trustees, Saturday 12th October 1935.

It was agreed on motion of Miss Whitton, seconded by Dr. Clark, to ask Dr. Farrell, Dr. Dwyer, and Dr. Jordan to interview Dr. Hendry and Dr. J.C. Connell and, at their discretion, other additional members of the Medical Faculty and report back to the meeting to be adjourned until 2 pm Sunday, October 13th, 1935.

This meeting of the Board of Trustees was duly assembled in Room 221, Douglas Library at 2 pm, Sunday, October 13th, 1935, with the following 20 members present.

The Chancellor, James A. Richardson, Esq. LL.D.

The Chairman, J.M. Macdonnell, Esq.

Dr. T.H. Farrell

The Principal, W.H. Fyfe, Esq., LLD

Hon. Senator H.H. Horsey

G.C. Bateman, Esq.

Dr. Dennis Jordan

Rev. G.A. Brown, DD.

D.H. Laird, Esq., KC

J.M. Campbell, Esq.

His Honour Judge Lavell

W.C. Clark, Esq. LLD

A.J. Meiklejohn, Esq.

Elmer Davis, Esq.

J.C. Macfarlane, Esq., KC

Dr. J.G. Dwyer

T.A. McGinnis, Esq.

J.M. Farrell, Esq. KC

Miss Charlotte Whitton, CBE

The Vice Principal, Dr. W.E. McNeill, serving as Secretary

A message was received from Mrs. Ross regretting her inability to be present.

Subject Cancer research

Dr. Dwyer on behalf of the Committee appointed at the meeting of October 12th submitted the following report.

After an extended discussion, Dr. Hendry Connell stated he was of the opinion that the following tentative procedure would meet with his views.

1. That the Hendry-Connell Foundation be turned over to the University to be designated as the HENDRY-CONNELL FOUNDATION OF QUEEN'S UNIVERSITY

2. That the stock of the Hendry Connell Foundation be turned over to the University

3. That the Patent or any Rights appertaining thereto be turned over to University or its nominee.

4. That Dr. Hendry Connell be appointed as Director of the Medical Research of the Hendry-Connell Foundation.

5. That the salary of the said Director be $10,000.00 for the first year, to be increased to $15,000.00 the second year, or as funds are available.

6. That a committee consisting of the following members:
   Dr. W.T. Connell
   J.M. Campbell
   J.M. Farrell
   Dr. J.C. Connell
   Dr. Hendry Connell
   Dr. James Miller
   Dr. L.J. Austin
   Dr. H. Farrell
   Dr. D. Jordan
   Dr. J.G. Dwyer
   Dr. McGhie, Deputy Minister of Health for Ontario
   Dr. Woodhouse, Deputy Minister of Health for Canada
   Dr. Fyfe, Principal, Ex Officio
   Shall be appointed by the trustees of the University
7. That the said committee crystallize the policies to be followed
   by the Hendry-Connell Foundation in all its aspects.

"It is tentatively understood that such committee shall handle all funds of the said Foundation, such funds to be earmarked for the said Foundation."

Dr. Dwyer stated that this report had been hurriedly prepared Sunday morning and was intended merely to give a general idea of the agreements. The phrasing in places was doubtless imperfect. In clause 3 above, for instance, he immediately agreed to add the words "or its nominee" which were not included in the report as submitted.

A lengthy discussion followed, and in reply to questions individual members of the committee gave their personal interpretations of various clauses.

Finally on a motion of Judge Lavell, seconded by the Principal, the following resolution was adopted:

"That the report be approved in principle and that it be referred to the Executive Committee to confer with the committee mentioned in the report and to recommend to the Full Board what further steps should be taken."

On motion of Mr. Davis seconded by Dr. Clark the meeting adjourned to be reconvened at the call of the Chairman.

In their report, the committee of three (appointed during the Saturday meeting 12th October 1935 to interview both Dr. J.C. and Dr. H.C. Connell), made no reference of Dr. J.C. Connell and referred only to an "extended discussion" with Dr. Hendry Connell, in their report to the Board of Trustees during the reassembly in Room 221 on Sunday October 13th, 1935.

On Monday October 14th, 1935 the Executive Committee met along with Dean Etherington of the Faculty of Medicine and Mr. King, University Solicitor, to consider their problem concerning the report of the committee of three presented to the board the previous day. The Executive Committee agreed to suggest certain modifications to the original proposal and asked a member, Mr. J.M. Campbell, to discuss these changes with the Connells prior to the conference planned with the committee that had been named on Sunday.

Mr. Campbell saw the senior Connell on Tuesday 15th October and was told that he and Dr. Hendry Connell were not prepared to enter into further discussion of the matter until they had time for consideration.

On Monday 21st October, 1935 Dr. J.C. Connell sent the following letter to Mr. J.M. Campbell representing Queen's University.

> Complying with your request during our conversation this morning I am giving you the following information relating to Hendry's affairs:
>
> 1. The proposals submitted by Doctors Dwyer, Farrell and Jordan were not accepted as a firm and binding arrangement but as a basis for new negotiations.
> 2. I heard nothing of the details proposed till after the meeting of the Board of Trustees but they were such as I could not advise Hendry to accept.
> 3. At our interview with you we stated that the proposals were not practical and asked that negotiations again be suspended.
> 4. We agreed not to accept any proposals which would take the research away from Kingston without giving Queen's a further opportunity to come to satisfactory terms.*

* It appears that Dr. J.C. Connell was trying to assure the Board of Trustees that Queen's would have equal control in the development of and research on Ensol. From the agreements reached, it would appear that these two points were understood by all involved.

5. An agreement has been made between the *Hendry-Connell Research Foundation and the Biochemical Research Foundation of the Franklin Institute, Philadelphia.*

6. The Franklin Institute is a strictly eleemosynary corporation, carrying on research in many departments of Science, without profit to any individuals.

7. The Franklin Institute has almost unlimited financial resources.

8. It has the best equipped cancer research personnel and laboratories in existence.

9. It is ready to assist in any way by advice, personal help and money to promote the necessary research on Hendry's problems to make the remedies available as soon as possible.

10. The Institute does not expect to be repaid in any way for money expended.

11. The Institute will be represented on the Board of the Hendry Connell Research Foundation by Dr. Ellis McDonald, Director of the Cancer Research Foundation and probably by Mr. Hayward, President of the Franklin Institute.

12. The patent rights for the United States will be assigned to the Franklin Institute which will look after the manufacture and distribution of the products in the United States.

13. Such plans will be agreed upon between the Hendry-Connell Research Foundation here and the Institute.

14. Ultimate profits from such operations will be entirely at the disposal of the Hendry-Connell Research Foundation. The Franklin Institute does not wish to share in them.

15. The Institute will spend $50,000.00 a year for the next three years, or more if necessary, to carry on the research in their laboratories in Philadelphia.

16. The Institute will give $25,000.00 to spend on research in Kingston each year for the next three years.

17. This money to be spent at the discretion of Dr. H.C. Connell.

18. This sum does not include any salary or honorarium for Dr. Connell.

19. The clinic necessary for clinical research will be continued at the General Hospital under the Foundation as at present.

20. Queen's University is asked to provide laboratory accommodation and service only.

21. It is intended to train and employ Canadian research workers as far as possible. Temporary assistance may be supplied from personnel in Philadelphia. Canadian workers may be asked to go to Philadelphia for training. When that is necessary the Institute is willing to pay expenses.
22. Dr. Connell and Mr. Holsgrove are invited to visit Philadelphia in the near future to see their equipment and meet the men doing the work.
23. The Franklin Institute will pay their expenses on this trip.

"It is my opinion that these plans are greatly to the advantage of the Hendry-Connell Research Foundation and also in the best interests of Queen's University. They insure a connection with one of the oldest research Institutes in the United States. The Franklin Institute was founded in 1824 and has always held the highest reputation for excellence of its work and for ethical standards. The motives of its present officials are beyond question and solely in the general interests of humanity.

Queen's will have only a minimum of expenditure to make, no commitments for the present or future, all the prestige of association with this important discovery and its development and the possibility of sharing in ultimate profits.

Laboratory accommodation to be provided at once will be temporary in character. Sooner or later a building specially adapted will be built. Some individual or corporation may be found to supply money for this purpose. The best site is proba-bly on the General Hospital grounds between the Laundry and the Nurses' Home."

Specific Proposal to Queen's University

1. The University will make the $4,000 already expended on the Connell Research a definite grant-without expectation of repayment.
2. The University will provide adequate laboratory accommodation for the Foundation and make any structural changes necessary without expense to the Foundation. It will further provide maintenance as follows:

Heat, twenty-four hours a day
Power
Gas
Services of special trades
Hot water and steam connections

3. The Hendry-Connell Research Foundation agrees to spend $25,000.00 a year for the next three years on research, paying all salaries and providing further equipment and general expenses.
4. At the end of three years this agreement may be reviewed and be terminated at any time with ninety days' notice.

These proposals with some minor alterations were agreed to, and planning was under way for construction of a suitable laboratory building on the hospital grounds.

That such a complete, concise and considered proposal should have been drafted by Dr. J.C. Connell should not have been any surprise to those board members who knew the man. He had led the Medical Faculty for 26 years as dean during its most formative and difficult years (1903 to 1929). For more than twenty-five years the senior Connell had been persuading and bullying where necessary, successive Boards of Trustees that they should serve the university with sense, energy and wisdom.

By early 1936, research was being carried on in the new laboratory situated on the hospital property at King Street West opposite the heating plant.

At the time the structure accommodated Ensol preparation, blood chemistry, cytology, private laboratories, dark room, storeroom and offices. The facility had been completed in record time. Dr. Ellis McDonald of the Franklin Institute had appointed a fully-trained bacteriologist and a blood chemist. By January, 1936, there were twenty-seven people in the employ of the Hendry-Connell Research Foundation. These included the clinical staff of full-time, part-time and consulting physicians, the trained laboratory workers, the technicians and the office personnel.

The plans and arrangements made in the fall of 1935 with Queen's University and The Franklin Institute permitted the work of the Hendry-Connell Research Foundation to go ahead with much less stress and considerably more professional assistance and interest.

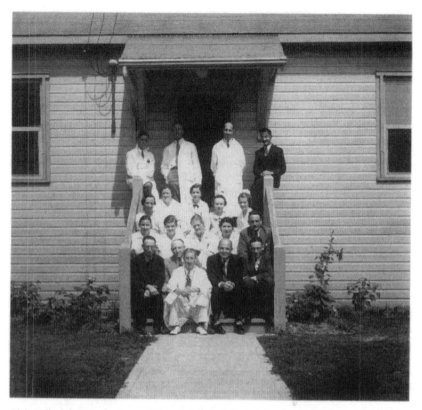

The staff of the Hendry-Connell Research Foundation at front entrance to new lab, King Street, Kingston, Ontario

There was a regular exchange of information between the Kingston and Philadelphia organizations.

Hendry was now receiving energetic help in carrying this work into the clinical field from these associates: Dr. C.D.T. Mundell; Dr. W.A. Jones; Dr. Charles Elliott; Dr. John Tweddell; Dr. John Delahaye; Dr. Fred Bonnell; Dr. I. Sutton and Dr. W.A. Campbell.

For guidance and consultation the following were always available for advice when requested: Dr. Alfred T. Bazin; Dr. James Miller; Dr. W.T. Connell; Dr. J.C. Connell; Dr. Harold Ettinger; Dr. L.J. Austin and Dr. Arthur L. Clark.

CHAPTER 4

The following bulletins have many case histories which are added to this story to show the types of patients and various geographical locations of those receiving the treatment.

There were three bulletins published in the years 1936-37-38.*

Bulletin No. 1 of the Hendry-Connell Research Foundation titled *Cancer Research* issued in August 1936 shows the following headings in the list of Contents:

CONTENTS OF BULLETIN NO.1

FOREWORD

LITERATURE SURVEY, BACTERIAL FILTRATES   *M.P. Munro*

STUDY AND TREATMENT OF CANCER BY PROTEOLYTIC ENZYMES (REPRINT)   *H.C. Connell*

SURVIVORS OF 29 CASES REPORTED UPON IN OCTOBER 1935

CLINICAL RESULTS IN ENSOL THERAPY   *H.C. Connell*

POST-MORTEM REPORTS OF CASES TREATED WITH ENSOL *James Miller* and *W.T. Connell*

HISTORIES OF SIXTEEN CASES OF CANCER TREATED WITH ENSOL IN AUSTRALIA   *Neville Davis*

HISTOLYTICUS STUDIES *Connell* and *Holsgrove*

BIO-CHEMICAL STUDIES OF BLOOD IN CANCER PATIENTS *F.B. Munro*

PRECIPITIN REACTIONS   *Connell* and *Holsgrove*

INTER-OCULAR ABSORPTION   *H.C. Connell*

REPORT TO NATIONAL RESEARCH COUNCIL (EXTRACT) CATARACT   *H.C. Connell*

This bulletin readily shows the range and the development of the work now that a proper base had been built.

* All these articles are available on request. See appendix.

We are printing here the Foreword from this bulletin, written by Hendry Connell, which explains its purpose and the future intentions of the Foundation.

This Bulletin is issued as a suitable medium for publication of information relating to the medical research work of the Foundation and of research which may be carried on in direct association with it.

In November, 1935, the Foundation became affiliated with the Biochemical Research Foundation of the Franklin Institute, Philadelphia of which Dr. Ellis McDonald is Director, for the special purpose of investigating the application of certain biological products to the treatment of cancer. Since December, 1935, there has been intimate collaboration of the work at the Foundations.

Bulletins will be published from time to time. This form is adopted to unite in one publication the laboratory and clinical aspects of research, to give coherence to the development of the various problems being studied and to afford those interested a complete account of results achieved.

SURVIVORS OF 29 CASES REPORTED UPON IN OCT. 1935

Case 2 Mrs. E.M., aged 45 years. The left ovary was removed on August 7, 1934, and found to contain papillomatous cysts which had involved the peritoneum. She was treated extensively with deep radiation following the operation.

On February 14, 1935, she was admitted to hospital complaining of severe crampy pelvic pain, constipation, bladder irritation, general cachexia and loss of weight.

Exploratory operation showed that the pelvis was matted with growth which had bound down the lower small intestine. Section of the growth was reported on as "secondary columnar cell carcinoma."

After discharge she was sent home to die. Morphia, 10 grs iv daily, was required to ease the pain. The bowels were very constipated and required enemata.

Treatment with Ensol was commenced May 14th as an experiment. An empirical dose of 2 cc was given every third day.

The patient steadily gained in weight, the bowels became normal, the appetite good. Opiates were reduced to heroin, gr 1/12, which has since been discontinued entirely.

On September 7th the patient appears a normal healthy individual. She is doing her own housework, going on picnics and swimming. No opiates are used; weight gain, 32 lbs. since May. The bowels are normal, no laxatives being necessary.

Case 8 Mr. W.C., aged 80 years. Previously reported. See reprint. This man was admitted to the medical wards on July 8, 1935. He complained of

1. Loss of appetite.
2. Loss of weight (60 lbs).
3. Weakness.
4. Vomiting.

The symptoms dated to about 3 months before admission. He gave a typical history of gastric trouble which was almost diagnostic. He noticed that he had small "gulping" vomiting about an hour after meals and every day or so, he had a huge ememis.

X-Ray examination of July 11th and histamine gastric analysis were both positive for cancer.

A surgical consultation suggested that operation was contraindicated by age and general condition.

He was started on Ensol treatment June 27th. By July 29th he had stopped vomiting, he was eating three ordinary meals a day and he had gained 3 lbs. in weight. Treatment was continued August 15th and his condition steadily improved. The mass in the abdomen entirely disappeared by September.

In October, patient caught cold and took to his bed. He became very feeble but continued to be free of all gastric symptoms up to his death on December 25th.

From August until December he received several short courses of treatment.

Case 10 Mrs. M., aged 61 years. Secondary carcinoma (proved at original operation) in both lungs, with osteoplastic and osteolytic changes in the upper lumbar vertebræ and suggestive changes in both hip bones and femurs. The original growth was in the left breast. Radical mastectomy in March, 1932, followed by routine deep radiation. She reported for treatment on July 21, 1935.

The patient was markedly breathless, even when at rest and had to be propped up in bed. On auscultation, there were marked changes in both lungs and fluid in both bases. This was later confirmed by X-ray. The heart was relatively normal. Her general condition was fair.

Treatment with Ensol was commenced on July 22, 1935. By the end of the first week the breathing had improved, so that patient could be comfortable when at rest. Improvement continued slowly until July 31st, when, after treatment, she had a sensation in the left chest and coughed up some dark phlegm. From this point on improvement was marked. On August 8th she was allowed to leave hospital and receive treatment as an out-patient. Breathlessness is apparent now only on exertion. She is taking gentle exercise and her general condition is improving.

Case 11 Mrs. L.W., aged 51 years. Carcinoma of the rectum; colostomy performed in 1931. She was fairly well until March, 1935, when a series of hæmorrhages occurred. Since then she has been going gradually down hill.

Treatment with Ensol was commenced on July 22nd. After five weeks' treatment her general condition has definitely improved and the rectal pain has eased.

Case 12 Mr. A.C., aged 57 years. A colloid carcinoma of ascending colon. An ileo-transverse colostomy was performed in June, 1935. This relieved the pain and obstructive symptoms but his general condition did not improve.

Treatment with Ensol was commenced on July 24th. After six weeks' treatment the man has gained 18 lbs. and has returned to part-time work.

Case 13 Mrs. A.H., aged 51 years. A malignant ulcer on the chest wall. The history began seven years ago. Both breasts have been removed. A recurrence in November, 1934, ulcerated and is now 8 1/2 by 5 inches at the widest points, with a typical rolled, raised, beaded edge. A mass of glands in the right supraclavicular region had involved the plexus, causing constant pain in the right arm.

Treatment was commenced on July 26th. On September 7th the

28

ulcer edges are flattened, the sides sloping and the base shows fresh granulation tissue. The arm pain is slightly relieved.

Case 14 Miss G.B., aged 56 years. Secondary metastases from an original scirrhous growth in the right breast, in the head of the 8th rib and in the body of the 7th dorsal vertebra. The spine was markedly angulated and she complained of constant pain, but there was no paralysis.

Treatment with Ensol was commenced on July 28th. The pain was controlled by August 7th. On August 29th the patient went home for a rest. The pain has not returned to date.

Case 15 Mr. F.C., aged 63 years. A mass in the bowel at the pelvi-rectal junction, adherent to the right side of the sacrum. Main complaints, pain over the sacrum and small thready stools. Cachexia is marked.

The case was diagnosed on July 25, 1935, and treatment with Ensol commenced on July 27th. The treatment continued to September 4th. The pain over the sacrum has lessened. The stools are larger and his colour is good. Appetite is fair and the weight has remained stationary.

Summary

Because of the very nature of this preliminary report it is impossible to discuss our clinical findings on a thoroughly scientific basis.

The cases have been treated and studied purely from the clinical point of view. Detailed biochemical examinations of the body fluids are being undertaken. Cytological studies of the cancer cells, comparing biopsy specimens before and after treatment, are being made and will be subsequently reported.

The solution has been used both intramuscularly and intravenously without any ill effects. Since but very little inert protein is present it produces no protein shock. We have experienced no allergic reactions.

The dosage is essentially individual. When pain is the predominating symptom the reaction dose produces a distinct increase in pain, commencing from one and a half to three hours after the intramuscular injection and lasting up to 24 hours, followed by complete disappearance. When the pain is not a feature of the case the reaction dose produces a "picking," or "pulling," sensation in the growth for the same period of time.

Most cases seem to respond after ten to fourteen days' treatment. In the group of cases at present under observation the effects are consistently good. There has been a marked gain in weight, with disappearance of severe cachexia. Visible growths have shown arrest, with softening and absorption. In the cases where pain has been a prominent symptom the sedatives have been cut in half and in many cases discontinued.

In the internal growths a similar process is apparently going on, since a great deal of clinical improvement has been noted.

It is altogether too soon to assess the ultimate value of the method. Weeks to months must elapse before we can determine if the cancer masses continue to show shrinkage and absorption till their complete disappearance. Clinical evidence so far leads us to think that such disappearance may occur.

Steps have been taken to prevent the exploitation of the public and the profession by unauthorized interests. Consequently, no supply of this solution will be made available until its value has been definitely proved.

The manufacture and therapeutic use of this enzyme solution is comparatively simple, when thoroughly understood. We can be responsible for no results obtained by investigators who have not had special training.

Much of the credit of carrying this work into the clinical field has been due to the energetic efforts of my esteemed associates, Dr. C.D.T. Mundell; Dr. W.A. Jones; Dr. Charles Elliott; Dr. John Tweddell; Dr. John Delahaye; Dr. Fred Bonnell; Dr. I. Sutton and Dr. W.A. Campbell.

For guidance and consultation I am indebted to Dr. Alfred T. Bazin, Dr. James Miller, Dr. W.T. Connell, Dr. J.C. Connell, Dr. Harold Ettinger, Dr. L.J. Austin and Dr. Arthur L. Clark.

For long and tedious laboratory assistance throughout the course of this investigation, I feel that a great deal of its success is due to the devoted service rendered by my technician, Mr. Bertram Holsgrove.

There are many others, too numerous to mention, who have given kind cooperation and assistance when it was most needed. To all these I extend my most sincere appreciation.

CLINICAL RESULTS OF ENSOL THERAPY
H.C. CONNELL

A year ago it was announced that a biological substance, probably an enzyme, had been discovered that appeared to arrest the growth of the cancer cell in the human body. That statement has been confirmed by biopsy, post mortem examination of tissues and by clinical results.

Intensive research has been carried on and is still in process upon the nature of the active substance, its standardization and its clinical effects. This paper deals with the clinical effects.

During the past year the Foundation has carried on a cancer research clinic at the Kingston General Hospital where the laboratory of the Foundation occupies a temporary building erected last November. Patients are admitted to the hospital as patients of the Foundation and are under the direct supervision of the clinical staff. There has been constant association between the laboratory and clinical staffs which contributes greatly towards progress in the research.

Over seven hundred patients have been registered. With few exceptions all have been referred by their own physicians to whom patients are returned with reports, and whose assistance has been given generously in after-care, treatment and observation. Over sixteen thousand individual doses have been given and not in any case has there been a generalized or allergic reaction nor any evidence that normal tissue has been damaged in any way.

With few exceptions cases treated have been far advanced in the progress of the disease. Most of them had received all that could be done by surgery, X-ray and radium. In this way the test of the value of Ensol treatment has been a severe one. Case histories are the final test of all this work.

As already stated, over sixteen thousand injections of Ensol have been made at the Kingston clinic alone and in no case was there any harmful reaction noted. On the other hand, in most of the cases it was evident that some important and beneficial change took place in the patient. It is clearly established that under this treatment cancer cells break down, liquefy and disappear. Biopsy and post mortem examination of tissues as well as clinical changes prove this to be the case. Recovery of the patient depends upon the extent of damage to tissue and function before the malignant process was arrested.

Biopsy and post mortem reports were done by Dr. James Miller and Dr. W.T. Connell.

A survey of all cases upon whom treatment was commenced, prior to May 1st, 1936, has been completed. Reports have been compiled up to the end of July, 1936. Any recent case that has not been under treatment for at least twelve weeks has not been included because it was felt that a mature judgment could not be formed as to the effects of Ensol.

This review has been carried out by an experienced clinician of over twenty-five years standing who is not in any way connected with this Research Foundation.

The files of 672 patients were examined, of which 184 were not treated for various reasons. The untreated cases can be grouped into moribund cases, those where metastasis was too generalized to offer any prospect of improvement, and, thirdly, where the diagnosis of cancer could not be established beyond doubt.

The remaining 488 patients were divided into two groups:-

1. 382 who received Ensol only, i.e., where not any surgery, radium or X-ray therapy had been employed within three months of the beginning of Ensol therapy.
2. 106 where Ensol was used either before or concurrently with surgery, radium or X-ray therapy in one or more combinations.

This review deals with the 382 cases who received Ensol only. Cases belonging to group (2) will be dealt with in a subsequent Bulletin. Biopsy confirmed the diagnosis of cancer in 367 out of the total 488 or a percentage of 74.4. Diagnosis in the remaining cases was made by a combination of X-ray, laparotomy and specialized instruments such as the oesophagoscope.

Reactions and Results

1. Pain is relieved.
2. Sensation is produced in the tumor mass.
3. Softening occurs in tumors.
4. Regression and disappearance of tumor.
5. Open lesions tend to heal.
6. Cachexia (ill state of body or mind) disappears.
7. Appetite returns or improves; gain in weight follows.
8. General feeling of well-being is restored.

These things occur in varying degree. If pain is present when Ensol is given it may be increased for a time and then disappear entirely. If no pain be present there may be some induced in and about the tumor for a variable period. In other cases there is a sensation of pricking or burning or merely a fullness or discomfort, depending on the site, extent and nature of the growth. Improvement of a general character may come on in a few days or may be delayed. With cessation of pain, narcotics, if in use, may be lessened or discontinued. Appetite returns and with improved metabolism, cachexia disappears and weight increases. Changes will be noted in the tumor mass if it is visible or palpable. It tends to become softer and smaller. Fixed masses become movable. Tenderness is lessened or disappears.

Too rapid softening or breaking down of the tumor mass may result in hæmorrhage. This may be avoided by adjustment of dosage.

There may well be a difference of opinion as to whether Ensol should be credited with producing the changes noted but when certain reactions take place with regularity in a great number of cases, cause and effect become firmly established, no matter how reluctant one may be to accept new ideas.

Pain Of the 382 cases pain was not a symptom of the disease in 88. Of the remaining 294, pain was partially or totally relieved in 279 cases, or 95%. In 15, the patients complained of increased severity of pain.

Softening and regression in tumor This occurred in 96 cases. This change could not be accurately determined in 103 cases because of the site of the cancer, e.g., stomach, bone, lung, liver. There were 279 cases where it was possible to observe this alteration in the tumor and 96 demonstrated positive evidence, or 34%.

Weight 97 patients gained weight from a few up to fifty pounds. This represents 25% of the cases treated but it is low because weight records were not always available.

Narcotics Diminution in the usage of narcotics followed relief of pain. In a great number of cases the employment of narcotics entirely ceased.

Conclusions

1. Ensol has been proved to affect beneficially late and advanced cases of cancer for which previously accepted methods of treatment have been totally ineffective.

2. It is premature to state how valuable Ensol will become as a therapeutic agent in cancer.
3. Ensol should be used in cancer in all stages, early and late. It must be left to the discretion of individual clinicians whether they will combine it with surgery, X-ray, and radium radiation.
4. Ensol, when employed preoperatively, has reduced in size and softened the growth.
5. Ensol should be employed postoperatively, in all cases.
6. Ensol should not be withheld in advanced cases where permanent changes are not likely. It will, in 95% of cases, palliate pain and render fatal termination less distressing.
7. In the 382 cases of this series the death rate was 47%. This figure may appear high but it must be realized that 53% of hopeless and abandoned cases are now alive.

Summary

1. Ensol contains an active principle which possesses the power to benefit proven cases of cancer by amelioration of symptoms and by partial or total disappearance of the growth.
2. The use of Ensol is free from any unpleasant reaction to the patient, local or constitutional – nor does it harm them in any way.
3. This series is too small and the period of time too short to draw any definite conclusion as to the ultimate value of Ensol, but it may be reasonably accepted that it does influence the course by partial or complete arrest in cases of advanced cancer.
4. The series is sufficiently large and the clinical improvement sufficiently constant to prove that the beneficial effect and regression in the growth observed, was not due to mere coincidence.
5. Ensol therapy was employed without any other therapeutic agent. Where radium or deep irradiation had been used treatment was not commenced until the radiologist admitted that no further improvement could be expected from his form of therapy. In many cases he stated that further irradiation would only aggravate the disease and cause increased pain.
6. Case 11 (scirrhus carcinoma of the breast) which had no other treatment, improved after one month's Ensol therapy to such a degree that the growth diminished by 75% with corresponding clinical improvement.

7. As in syphilis and other constitutional diseases one course of Ensol therapy will not suffice but repeated courses will be necessary for the continuance of the beneficial influence of Ensol on cancer.

It is not premature to express the hope that the early publication of Dr. Hendry Connell's continued laboratory work will lead to a wider recognition of the great value of this new therapeutic agent. If employed in cases of cancer in all stages (early or advanced) both in conjunction with and separate to other known methods it will lead to a lowering of the cancer mortality rate, which has not been influenced during the past decade.

BULLETIN

OF THE

HENDRY-CONNELL
RESEARCH FOUNDATION

NO. 2

CANCER RESEARCH

JANUARY, 1937

KINGSTON, ONT. CANADA

CONTENTS OF BULLETIN NO. 2*

LABORATORY NOTES

It is intended that the next issue of the Bulletin will contain mainly reports of progress in the work of the laboratory.

The results of further studies of Histolyticus are now ready for publication.

The method of standardizing Ensol filtrates is completed and may be reported soon.

Investigation of the blood chemistry of cancer patients before and during treatment with Ensol points toward a means of diagnosis and prognosis.

Study is also being made of the action of the blood serum of cancer patients on cancer tissue substrate, before and during treatment with Ensol.

*All these articles are available on request. See appendix.

An appeal is made to surgeons and pathologists to forward cancer tissue to the Kingston Laboratory. All available tissue from the operating table or autopsy room can be used for the manufacture of Ensol and for extension of the laboratory studies. Tissue comes safely from a point as far distant as Vancouver. Containers are provided and all expenses paid. Anyone willing to assist will please write to the Foundation for instructions.

ENSOL

H.C. CONNELL, BA, MD, CM

This is an effort to answer questions asked by visitors and contained in letters from physicians.

What is Ensol?

The fundamental discovery is that of a biological product which can be injected into the human body without harm, and which appears to exert a profound influence upon malignant growth.

If that is true and the observations of the past eighteen months continue to be confirmed in a constantly widening field, Ensol needs no advocate. It will make its way despite skepticism, suspicion, personal interest or barrage of abuse.

If it is not true, no advocate can prevent or even postpone its disappearance into the limbo of forgotten nostrums.

It is not a "one man" exploit or undertaking. More than sixty people, biochemists, bacteriologists, cytologists, physicists, clinicians, at the two Foundations, are working on the problems opened out by this discovery.

Investigations in laboratory and clinic are being correlated and, in both, will need to go on indefinitely. Physicians everywhere who may use Ensol are invited to report their results whether they be positive or negative. Case histories should be made as complete as possible. The Bulletin will always be open for such reports.

Ensol is not a "cure."

It does not produce typical reactions and results in all cases in which it is administered.

Its present limitations are fully recognized, acknowledged and accepted.

Ensol is a research problem upon which intensive coordinated work is being done, in laboratories and clinics.

Definite clinical results are being obtained by its use, so definite that general use is warranted as soon as possible.

These definite results are being secured not only at the original clinic but at many different places under varying conditions and by competent independent observers.

Ensol is a filtrate produced by the action of a non-pathogenic proteolytic micro-organism on cancer tissue.

Protein is obtained from cancer tissue by separating it from other constituents.

The organism is seeded on this protein and incubated for a variable time.

The liquids and solids are then separated by centrifuge. The liquid portion is filtered through a Berkefeld candle to make it sterile.

The resulting filtrate contains an active substance probably an enzyme, which is now called Ensol (en zyme sol ution).

The exact nature of the active substance is not known.

It is assumed to be an enzyme.

It has been separated from certain other constituents of the solution but not isolated.

Solutions have been standardized for clinical use.

About one hundred and twenty-five physicians have had the use of Ensol from the Kingston laboratory, without charge.

A large amount has also been supplied, gratis, to physicians from the affiliated laboratory at Philadelphia.

How is Ensol administered?

It is injected into the muscles. It can be given intravenously.

No advantage has been noted from intravenous use.

It is to be administered by the physician himself.

Dosage determined by the effect produced from day to day.

What does Ensol do?

Over twenty-five thousand injections have been given to patients at the Kingston clinic alone. In no case has there been any harmful reaction.

There is no clinical or post mortem evidence that it is harmful to normal tissues or functions.

It does not produce a reaction elevation of temperature.

It does arrest the growth of the cancer cell in the human body.

It produces a sensation in the tumor mass.

It relieves pain and tenderness.

Cachexia disappears.

Appetite returns or improves.

There is a gain in weight.

A general feeling of well being is restored.

Softening of tumors is noted.

Fixed masses become movable.

Regression and disappearance of tumors take place.

Open lesions tend to heal.

Narcotics, if in use, are reduced in quantity and may be discontinued entirely.

Naturally, these things occur in varying degree and in some cases not at all.

When should Ensol be used?

It is not suggested or intended that the use of Ensol should replace presently accepted methods of treatment. Rather it should be added to them.

There is no contraindication for its use.

It should be used in every case of malignant growth and as soon as possible.

On what classes of cases has Ensol been used?

1. Cases diagnosed malignant which refused surgery and/or radiation.
2. Early cases which had surgery and/or radiation, the use of Ensol being added in the hope of assisting in prevention of extension or recurrence.
3. Cases diagnosed malignant, clinically or by biopsy, pronounced inoperable and not suitable for radiation and regarded as hopeless.
4. Cases upon which all the resources of surgery and radiation had been employed and then pronounced incurable and hopeless.

There are illustrations of all these in the case histories related in this Bulletin. The majority of cases treated fall into categories 3 and 4, as Ensol at the present time is a last resort for those who have been informed that the resources of surgery and radiation have been exhausted on their behalf and they must face the future without hope. As soon as Ensol is available for general use cases will probably receive it in earlier stages with greater average benefit.

ENSOL AT PORTLAND, MAINE
Treatment of Seven Cases of Cancer with Ensol (Rex)
W.H., MD
Portland, Maine

Rex is the temporary name given to Ensol made in the laboratories of the Biochemical Research Foundation of the Franklin Institute, Philadelphia, which is affiliated with the Hendry-Connell Research Foundation, Kingston. Dr. H was supplied from the laboratory in Philadelphia.

Clinical Reports on Patients Treated by Rex

Patient (F.H.H.) Age 70; occupation, Blacksmith; Address, Norway, Maine.

History Was referred to me by Dr. E.K. of West Paris, Maine. Said that the patient complained of being sick to the stomach with some pain, poor appetite, short of breath, nocturia ten to twelve times, and a loss of 44 pounds in weight. Onset of symptoms one year ago.

Examination Upon examination found Mr. H. emaciated with a loud diastolic murmur in his heart, decompensated and rather harsh breathing at the base of his lungs.

An X-ray by Dr. P. of the Sisters Hospital in Lewiston was said to have shown metastatic malignancy of the spine with a primary focus in the pancreas. That his stomach was displaced upward with considerable widening of the duodenal loop. No gross obstruction. The mass displacing stomach is pancreas and definitely enlarged.

Mr. H. was rather a difficult patient to treat, absolutely refusing to have any surgery done. On palpation in the region of his pancreas was a tumor the size of an ordinary orange. The prostate was very suggestive of carcinoma.

He was started on Rex, using No. 28 and followed by No. 22. (These numbers are vials of Rex made from different tissue).

No examination of the tumor was done for four or five days, when as a matter of interest his abdomen was palpated. Much to my surprise there was no tumor to be felt, his nausea was considerably better and in a few days he was able to eat without throwing it up.

Feeling that prostate was the origin of the trouble, Mr. H. was prevailed upon to be admitted to the Maine General Hospital on April 4th for X-ray pictures of his chest and pelvis. The impression rendered by the radiologist was as follows:

Pelvis
I believe that the probability is that the increased density and particularly in the region of the pubic bones, is due to metastatic malignancy from the carcinoma of the prostate.
Chest
The increased density as seen in the bones of the chest and clavicles is rather suggestive of metastatic malignancy. However, it is possible that it could be due to Paget's disease.

Because of the fact that the patient was suffering from bladder irritation it was suggested that radon implants be used in an effort to shrink down the prostate, in the meantime continuing Rex. On April 4th, 12 non-removable radon seeds were implanted in his prostate in the hopes of palliation. In a week the irritation of the bladder was markedly improved, whether due to radon or Rex it is impossible to determine. The patient was improving and it was advised that he return home to convalesce, thinking he would live during the summer. On April 15th he was suddenly taken with a chill, rapid rise in temperature, and he expired April 16th from bilateral lobar pneumonia.

Summary In this case there was definite and marked relief following the use of Rex. It was too much to expect the treatment to cure such an advanced case, but I feel that the palliation would have been very much worth while had not pneumonia stepped in and claimed its victim.

Patient (E.T.) Age 66; Freeport, Maine.
History Two months ago thought he had piles. There was bleeding once in a while and the bowel movements poor. There was no pain but a pressing down feeling. His appetite is good but he has lost some weight.
Examination Annular carcinoma of the rectum just inside the anus and extends upward for 4 or 5 inches.

On December 28th a colostomy was done and during the operation it was demonstrated that there were no apparent pelvic glands or involvement of the rectum above the limits already referred to.

Rex was started January 3rd, using routine dosage of initial 1/3 cc and increasing the dosage 1/3 of a cc daily. The last two were small amounts of approximately 5 cc in each vial.

On February 5th his colostomy was working well. Patient stated that he felt well, was gaining strength and weight and there was no bleeding from his rectum. On March 4th colostomy was fine, the tumor in the rectum still present and could just admit the index finger in its lumen.

Summary This patient had an inoperable, annular adenocarcinoma of the rectum. Colostomy performed and the following Rex treatments given in two series.

No ill effects at any time. No marked improvement of the cancer itself could be demonstrated except that there was no bleeding. Patient complained of pain at no time. To date have had no complaints from this patient who has not been seen since May.

Examined September 1st, 1936, and no apparent improvement. Patient failing slowly.

Patient (G.F.)-Age 69; occupation, Farmer; Sterling Junction, Mass.
History January 23, 1935, had a colostomy by Dr. C. of Boston at The New England Baptist Hospital. There was so much involvement of the rectum by the carcinoma that it was impossible to resect the colon. When examined by me December 10, 1935, colostomy was working most satisfactorily. The rectum just filled the pelvis and was causing obstruction to urination by pressure on the bladder. The rectum bled easily and there was a bloody mucous discharge from the anus which made it necessary for him to sit down whenever he urinated. Patient was suffering considerable pain, had difficulty in passing his water and urination was followed by a great deal of discomfort. Had lost some weight.

Treatment was begun December 10, 1935, using Rex, the dosage taken 1/3 cc and the dose increased 1/3 of a cc daily. On December 14 and 15 patient admitted no improvement. On December 18 a new bottle of Rex used. On the 19th patient complained of some nausea, was put on liquid diet and given no treatment. On the 20th, patient said he had some pain during the night but had no nausea. Treatment resumed. On the 21st, patient volunteered that he had urinated during the night without pain for the first time. On the 22nd had taken a laxative and the colostomy kept him up for more than two hours. On the 26th patient was unable to receive his treatment because of   my personal incapacity. On the 31st patient received his final dose amounting to 5 cc and his parting remark was: "I am convinced that I have been helped.

I have much less pain; I am able to sleep better; I pass my water easier and with much less discomfort and I have no bleeding or discharge from the rectum."

Patient was advised that at the end of three or four weeks if he was convinced he had been helped and wished to take a second series I considered it advisable.

On January 17, 1936, Mr. F. felt that he had been helped enough to take another series of treatment. This treatment was delayed until Feb. 11 due to lack of supply of Rex. On February 11 he returned for treatment which was begun with Rex. His complaint was that the pain had begun to come back and was having some trouble with his urine but neither was as bad as it was at first before he had begun the first series of Rex. On the 14th complained of having had a bad night with pain and difficulty with his urine. On February 15 Rex. On the 15th he made the statement that for two days he had felt kind of mean with a little nausea and headache but that today he felt excellent. Except for pain in the end of his penis was feeling very well. On February 27: "can truthfully say I am better. Have had two good nights and I take fewer pain pills." On the 24th he was still feeling better and the pain in his bladder was a great deal less. On March 20 he went to his local doctor and made the statement that he had had definite relief from his previous treatment, that he still had some poor days, some pain in the morning after getting up but that he would take one tablet every four hours during the day and none at night and could go twelve hours and be comfortable even at the end of twelve hours. Looks very well and returned voluntarily for his third series of Rex treatment.

On March 20. A 1/2 cc dose was given. No reaction. On the 21st Rex was used. This series was given without anything remarkable to report and the patient returned to his home. He has recently asked for a fourth series which up to the present time has not been given because of lack of Rex with which to treat him.

Summary Patient was hopeless and had been given up by his surgeon. Disease was cancer of the rectum filling his entire pelvis and involving the bladder. Treatment was by Rex as follows:

Rex, dated 11- 5-35.
Rex, dated 12- 6-35.
Rex, dated 1-12-36.
Rex, dated 1-27-36.

Rex, dated 1-21-36.

Rex, No. 28.

Rex, No. 22.

Marked palliation obtained. Patient still living and desirous of further treatment.

Patient (W.F.)-Age 30; South Bristol, Maine; admitted to the Maine General Hospital December 31, 1935, discharged January, 1936; occupation, Letter Carrier.

The patient was first admitted to the hospital October 26, 1935, and discharged November 13, 1935.

History About ten weeks previous to his admission on October 26, he developed low back ache. No stomach distress. At this time noticed small gland in the posterior chain on the left side of his neck. This has remained stationary. Three weeks prior to admission had another severe back ache and cervical glands increased in size. No soreness or tenderness; his appetite was good. No nausea or vomiting. No loss of weight, but has been feeling tired. Examination at this time showed posterior chain glands enlarged on the left side, hard and not tender. There was a healed scar over the posterior glands, the anterior chain enlarged. Glands on the right side palpable. Thyroid not palpable. No tracheal tug. The X-ray of chest not enlarged. On the left there is a suspicion of enlargement. Lumbar spine and pelvis and abdomen are otherwise negative. On Nov. 6 and 9 gastro-intestinal X-ray gave the impression of normal oesophagus, stomach and duodenum, but there was a slight irregularity of the fundus which seemed to disappear after the stomach filled. There was occult blood in the stool. Wasserman and Kahn tests negative. The biopsy was made of gland removed from the neck. Careful study of the sections revealed colloid material and it was finally decided that the carcinomatous gland arose from the thyroid. The blood analysis showed a moderate anemia, but otherwise negative. Patient was given deep X-ray therapy and discharged to his local doctor.

Upon his second admission, that is December 31, 1935, the patient has been up and about and was able to go out gunning. Suffered no pain, but 13 days ago commenced to have pain in his bowels and about his navel, and his constipation has increased during the past ten or twelve days. Has had three enemas a day for the last five days without very good results. His appetite is poor and he has considerable indigestion. On January 3, 1936, gastro-intestinal X-ray examination gave the impression of an abdominal mass in relation to the duodenum which caused partial obstruction from pressure, but no stricture. The X-ray examination of the chest shows a marked increase in the hilus region which is considerably more than in the previous film taken October 29, 1935; and distributed throughout both lung fields are irregular areas of increased density which were not present on the film taken October 29. These are undoubtedly general metastatic areas of both chests. The patient was seen at a clinic by Dr. S.W. who gave a most unfavorable prognosis. The patient was discharged from the hospital on January 4, 1936.

On January 8th, 1936, Mr. F.'s doctor, Dr. F. of Pemaquid, called up and said that the patient was failing rapidly and, having heard of Dr. Connell's Ensol treatment, asked if it would be possible as a last resort to try it on Mr. F. Mr. F's mother came into see me and after explaining to her there was no definite assurance that Mr. F. would be helped by Ensol but that, if he and she wished to try it, there being no charge for the Ensol, I said that I would be willing to give it to him. Although Mr. F. was very weak, under opiates he was able to be brought from South Bristol to Yarmouth, where he is stopping with his sister. A trained nurse accompanied him (Mrs. C.). The patient was seen by me January 9th. He was very emaciated, extremely jaundiced, suffering abdominal pain, considerable spasm over the upper abdomen consistent with the areas over the gall bladder and pancreas. The patient was nauseated and vomited and could not take any solid food. Ensol was started on the morning of January 9th, 1936.

The Rex was given as usual starting with 3/10 of a cc and increasing daily 3/10 until 21 treatments had been given, dated 11-25-35, dated 12-30-35, dated 1-20-36, dated 2-3-36

The following notations:
Jan. 9th, spasm over the gall bladder and cardiac end of the stomach probably pancreatic in origin.

Jan. 11th, was seen by his physician, Dr. F., who stated that his appearance was greatly improved.

Jan. 12th, very yellow and pain in his testicle.

Jan. 25th, lemon yellow.

Jan. 26th, pain in the left kidney region.

Jan. 27th, definite improvement. Felt some discomfort for two or three hours after treatment.

Jan. 30th, looks much better, has been able to eat without vomiting for several days, says he feels pretty well and what pain he has is in the left lower quadrant.

Feb. 2nd, was very yellow again and liver dullness 3 and 4 inches below the costal margin. However, the patient feels pretty well.

Feb. 13th, patient looks bad, sore throat, some cough, can feel nodular liver 3 inches below the costal margin.

Patient died Feb. 22nd.

Summary This patient was suffering from extensive metastasis throughout chest, abdomen and liver, the origin being carcinoma of the thyroid. He had received extensive X-ray therapy and was sent home to die Jan. 4th, 1936. Absolutely hopeless case and the patient so bad on Jan. 9th that he could not even reach the hospital, yet the improvement was so marked and definite following the use of Rex that the family in their delight reported the patient as being cured. Here again palliation was sufficient to be of distinct encouragement.

Nurses Notes
Jan. 9th, 1936-Patient fairly comfortable but very weak; color poor; skin jaundiced; eyes yellow; lips pale; appetite poor; dull pain in lumbar region. Severe pain in lower back. Sleeping-10 p.m.

Jan. 10th, 1936-Patient slept well entire night. Slight pain in lower left back; color sallow; lips dry and pale; pulse rapid and strong; patient weak. Urine concentrated; dark and cloudy. Appetite poor. Severe pain in back and thighs. Awake-no pain but general stiffness. Severe pains in lower back and thighs. Sleeping-10 p.m.

Patient Mrs. H.H.-Age 41; Portland, Maine.

Diagnosis Epidermoid carcinoma of the cervix, Group IV, rapidly growing.

History First seen May 13th, 1935. Had a history of irregular bleeding for three years and had been bleeding steadily for eight weeks. Had been under the care of a physician who told her he was building her up so that something could be done. She was taken to the Maine General Hospital in an ambulance where two transfusions were given and the patient treated with radium. There was an enormous everting growth of the cervix with considerable involvement of the vaginal wall on the left, both broad ligaments and the pelvis frozen. In June patient recovered so that she was able to take a series of deep X-ray therapy and by

August the local condition had cleared up nicely but there was extension of the growth up under the bladder and into the left wall of the vagina. This was treated with radium seeds. In September, 1935, patient was feeling fine with no pain or ache at all and was about town. In November patient was having a good deal of pain in the bladder and especially in the back, left side of bladder, left thigh and left big toe.

Rex treatment was begun November 30, routine dosage starting with 1/3 cc and increasing 1/3 cc daily being carried out. The first three days patient complained of increased pain following injection. On December 3 she had no discomfort whatsoever. On December 9th a second ampule of Rex was used. On the 10th complained of some discomfort for a while although there was no pain in the right hip. On December 13th patient was out of bed and entirely comfortable except in the region of the bladder. December 15th the bladder condition much improved. December 16th had characteristic rheumatic pain in the shoulders, knees and hips. On the 17th discomfort in the bladder and rectum a great deal less, appetite good, patient up and dressed. Thinks she is decidedly better and treatment discontinued for two weeks. On December 29th a vaginal examination shows that the vaginal growth had smoothed up a great deal. The growth in the left fornix is contracted, is smooth although hard, the pain in the back is gone, much less in the bladder and hardly any in the left leg or big toe. On January 4th was called to see the patient who was having a good deal of pain in the region of the bladder on the left side and was passing some blood in the urine. When the small clots of blood were passed by the urethra it was very painful and the passing was followed with considerable discomfort. A second series of Rex started, this series was continued until February 11th. On January 25th had been passing for several days clots of blood from the bladder with considerable pain. On the 27th patient felt a good deal better. On the 29th the urine still bloody but quite comfortable and eating a little more. On February 11th, dated 2-3-36. The urine is clearer and the clots are fewer. Patient failing quite rapidly. Expect her to live but a few days. Patient died February 18th. Was conscious for several days, apparently in no pain and had no morphine during the last week of illness.

Summary A hopeless case to begin with. Was given:

Rex
dated 11-22-35
dated 11-5-35

dated 12-30-35

dated 1-20-36

dated 2-3-36 (In this only one or two doses given.)

No ill effects from any treatment given and decided palliation obtained which I feel certain was due to use of Rex.

Patient E.D.-Age 82; Worcester, Mass.

History For 5 or 6 years, Mrs. D. has concealed a scirrhous carcinoma of the breast. Last August it was a bleeding, sloughing mass with extensive involvement in the axilla, the skin of the axilla being perforated in 5 or 6 different places. A simple mastectomy was performed in order to get rid of the sloughing mass. Some radium was used in the axilla. The patient returned to Worcester and there tried to conceal the fact that she had been operated upon or had any lesion whatsoever. In November she was brought to the Maine General Hospital in Portland apparently dying from old age or carcinomatosis. X-ray didn't show any involvement of the lungs or bones. She was given two deep X-ray treatments but became so nauseated that she refused to take any more. The pectoralis major muscle was swollen, hard, and the axilla was one hard mass with a sloughing center. It was necessary to dress this two and three times a day. There was a great deal of pain and the patient was expected to die.

On November 24th treatment was begun with Rex, the dose as usual beginning with 1/3 cc and increasing it daily. On November 28th there was a marked improvement in the lesion. The pectoralis major had softened, the redness had gone out of it, the discharge from the axilla was negligible and the mass itself had softened and there was no discomfort whatsoever. Treatment was continued until December 2. Treatment was stopped because it was apparent that the patient was about through. Patient died December 3rd. For several days the patient had not eaten, was nauseated, was free from pain and was delirious.

Summary The primary cause of death was inanition, arteriosclerosis, psychosis. Secondary, scirrhous carcinoma of the breast with extension into axilla.

Patient Mrs. N.M. Age 44; Portland, Maine.

History In June, 1935, was treated for carcinoma of the cervix by Dr. A.P.L.

Complaint Pain in both legs and thighs, very tired. At present is a morphine addict; is luetic.

Examination No bleeding visible, cervix nodule, hard, unhealthy in appearance. Both broad ligaments involved and pelvis frozen. Patient had series of deep X-ray treatments in September. In November was called to see patient at her home. Found her in bed unable to be up because of pain in her pelvis and as above mentioned an addict of morphine. Rex treatment promised her if she would cooperate in leaving off opiates. It was necessary to call in the federal inspector in order to shut off different sources of supply.

Rex treatment was started November 21st and given daily to December 3rd when there was interval owing to lack of Rex solution until December 9th, when the treatment was resumed, the dosage as is given routinely, starting with 1/3 cc and increased the daily dosage 1/3 of a cc until 5 cc's are given.

Notes First day of treatment patient complained of a picking sensation in the pelvis. The second day complained of a lot of pain. The third day was quite comfortable. The fourth day considerable discomfort probably due to overdose of laxative. Is also cutting down on the morphine. On the 26th of November received no treatment and had taken but 2 1/2gr of morphine in the last 24 hours. On the 27th apparently improved. Some pain in the back but thinks it is better. On November 30th, after having had 9 treatments, was up about the room, telephoning; had received one or two sterile hypos with fair results. On December 1st says there is pain about 1 1/2 hours after injection. No treatment from December 3rd until December 9th because of lack of solution. December 10th says she is having pain but not from the injection. December 12th up and dressed and walked quarter of a mile to the grocery store. On December 13th was in my office for a treatment. On December 15th condition quite satisfactory. December 16th no opiates. On the 17th stole three sodium amytal tablets. Was up at 8 o'clock and active, had no complaints, drove 70 miles to Bethel, Maine, and has had a good appetite for two or three weeks. On December 21st, four or five days after treatment stopped, patient found at home in a state of unconsciousness due to several allonal pills. Husband was drunk and the house a wreck. Patient was taken to the psychopathic hospital but due to misunderstanding and complications was released. Patient's statements have to be somewhat discounted because of drug habit and some of the pain may be due to luetic lesions of the cord. At present I am having nothing to do with this patient until she voluntarily clears up her addiction to drugs. My impression is that this patient was helped considerably so that she was able during the series of treatment to leave a sick bed and be about town with very little discomfort. The improvement in weight and diet also points to benefit derived from the treatment. Patient continued her drug habit and began to hemorrhage from the cervix and died June 6, 1936.

ENSOL AT VANCOUVER GENERAL HOSPITAL

H.C.P., MD

Pathologist to the Hospital

Over one hundred and seventy-five cases of cancer have been treated with Ensol at the Vancouver General Hospital since October, 1935. The following are histories of fifteen of these cases selected to indicate what may be expected to occur with the treatment. The Ensol used was supplied from the laboratory of the Hendry-Connell Foundation at Kingston.

H.P., male, 63 Had transurethral prostatic resection in 1933 and extensive deep X-ray therapy since. Past few months cough, sciatic pain, occasional bloody sputum and pain in chest. Began Ensol treatment Oct. 5, 1935, and was given 2 courses of 20 injections and 4 of 10 each. He experienced definite relief of pain during the greater part of treatment, but had several semi-collapses, evidently myocardial in origin, during his course of treatment. His malignancy gradually progressed and he died in April, 1936. However, he seemed generally more comfortable during treatment than previous to starting it.

J.F, male, 61 yrs. Frequency of urination with burning began in July 1935. By October had incontinence and prostate was found enlarged and firm. TUPR done with diagnosis of carcinoma. Began Ensol treatment Jan. 6th, 1936, at which time the prostate was firm, almost sclerotic and the size of a golf ball. Has had 6 courses of treatment and although prostate enlarged gradually, till at present time it is the size of a large hen's egg, it is softer, patient feels better, has no nocturia and has gained weight. Has very occasional slight streaking of blood at termination of urination.

Mrs. D.C. age 32 First noticed lump in left breast Jan., 1932, accompanied by pain of a "continuous, pricking, shooting dragging" type. Treated by osteopath for 3 mos., then consulted physician. Breast amputated in Aug., 1932, with post operative X-ray for 12 mos. In March, 1934, recurrence, old site; treated with radium and mass disappeared. In Sept., 1935, recurrence, same area, lost 14 lbs. in one year. Reported for Ensol treatment Nov. 20th, 1935, and on examination shows a small navel orange sized mass in midportion of scar in left breast. It is reddish-blue in color but not ulcerated and very firm. The surrounding tissue is rather indurated and somewhat congested; this may be due to the previous X-ray and radium therapy. A few small pea-sized nodules are present in the adjacent skin. Began Ensol treatment Nov. 20th and one week after beginning treatment a serous oozing from the mass in the scar was noted. A few days later this became bloody and within 6 weeks the mass was definitely smaller and showed well marked sloughing. Smaller nodules in the skin show marked softening. Gained 4 lbs. in first two months. Occasional bleeding from growth and it became much more necrotic and foul-smelling and it was felt that X-ray therapy might help to destroy this sloughy mass and in July, 1936, was given 10 treatments with the desired result. Has had 7 courses of Ensol and at present time shows a deep, fairly clean ulcer at previous site of growth. The skin nodules are smaller. Patient's weight has been maintained and no axillary or other glands can be noted.

Mrs. H.R. age 49 years From Oct., 1933, noticed that the abdomen was gradually enlarging. Frequency of urination and irregular menses. In Dec., 1935, consulted physician who diagnosed ovarian tumor and a right ovarian carcinoma of papillary type was removed. Six months later, an abdominal paracentesis was done and again 6 mos. after this. Began Ensol treatment in March, 1936, and has definite lobulated firm masses in lower abdomen, bilateral, and some fluid. Has had 5 courses of Ensol and there has been no increase in size of abdomen and patient says she feels definitely better while taking Ensol. Weight has been practically stationary.

J.M.-male, age 49 History of gastric ulcer, also left lower quadrant pain, constipation and diarrhoea, 7 yrs., and after medical ulcer treatment was operated and a large ulcer near esophagus was found, artificially perforated and repaired. Had return of ulcer symptoms in about 7 mos. and was put on medical treatment again. Was in hospital in Sept., 1934, and Jan., 1935. LLQ pain has become very severe with obstructive symptoms, blood and mucus in stool. Proctoscopic examination showed obstructing carcinoma, rectum. Laparotomy showed it to be inoperable and a colostomy was performed, followed by X-ray treatment. Began Ensol treatment Oct. 28th, 1935. Prior to this, had been taking morph. gr 1/6 every 4 hrs., but after one week's treatment reduced this to 1/6 at night only. For approximately 8 mos. since beginning Ensol treatment, has been relatively comfortable with, however, occasional bouts of abdominal pain and diarrhoea, but color has remained good and he has maintained weight. In June, 1936, was admitted to hospital with severe lower abdominal pain, possibly due to some obstruction of colostomy. Barium enema shows none, however. Any operative interference was considered unwise and he was put on sedatives, etc., and Ensol treatment continued. He had alternating periods of moderate comfort, pain and diarrhoea from this time until his death, Oct. 20th, 1936. He had 7 courses of Ensol in all and I believe was made fairly comfortable during its use.

J.M.-male, age 67 Weakness, pallor, shortness of breath, pain in small of back and between shoulders for the past 9 mos. Has a number of firm enlarged glands, left axilla. Is rather emaciated, anaemic and findings are relatively negative with the exception of left axillary glands, one of which was excised and reported microscopically as carcinoma of, possibly, bronchiogenic origin. X-ray of the chest-possible old pneumoconiosis, though possibility of mediastinal tumor. Began Ensol treatment Sept. 27, 1935, and has had 3 courses; one of 20 and two of 10 injections. Patient gained some weight, felt better, color improved and there is definite softening of the glands in the left axilla. Pain and shortness of breath ameliorated definitely during treatment. Patient is still alive (Nov. 16, 1936) but suffering chiefly from cerebral arteriosclerosis at present.

Mrs. F.S., age 53 Excision of tumor in rt. breast 1 mo. before applying for Ensol treatment. Microscopic diagnosis, adenocarcinoma. Refused even simple mastectomy, X-ray or radium therapy. Began Ensol treatment Nov. 1st, 1935. Has gained 10 lbs. in weight. Feels and looks well and examination to-day, Nov. 18th, 1936, reveals no palpable evidence of recurrence in breast or axilla. Has had 3 courses of Ensol; one of 20 and two of 10 injections.

Mrs. A.C., age 40 Loss of weight, abdominal enlargement, menorrhagia 3 mos., general weakness. Laparotomy Feb. 1st, 1935, 4 qts. bloody fluid in abdomen. Left and right ovaries completely replaced by massive papillary carcinomatous growth which also involved omentum, visceral and parietal peritoneum. Diagnosed as cystadenoma papilliform malignum. Began Ensol treatment Sept. 24th, 1935. Abdomen decreased 4" in circumference within 3 weeks after institution of Ensol therapy and patient seemed stronger and brighter until about one month after treatment began, developing left hydrothorax which was aspirated with great relief to patient. About one week after this she died suddenly from an acute cardiac dilation.

Mrs. F.L., age 53 Diarrhoea 2 yrs. Loss of weight (12 lbs. in 2 yrs.). No blood in stools, considerable mucus; occasional vomiting. Poorly nourished, nervous woman; no definite palpable masses found on examination. Gastro-intestinal series revealed an extensive encephaloid appearing carcinoma, middle 1/3 of stomach which was considered inoperable. Began Ensol treatment and there was definite abatement of the diarrhoea. Had 7 courses of Ensol and during the past months almost continuous injections, i.e., every 3 or 4 days. Said she felt much better, while taking Ensol, and there seemed to be definite amelioration of the diarrhoea during this time. However, she began to regress during the past few weeks and died a little over one year after beginning treatment.

C.B., male, age 24 Recurrence of tumors in muscles of left leg during past 8 yrs. Recurring after excision. Has had deep X-ray therapy over this area and whole left lower extremity. Only point of interest in examination is the presence of 4 fairly firm masses in the peroneal tendon sheaths of the left leg. They were excised, Jan. 31st, 1936, and found to be fairly well circumscribed, although one was firmly adherent of the periosteum of fibula. Microscopic diagnosis: fibromyxosarcoma. Began Ensol treatment Feb. 25th, 1936. Has had 5 courses of Ensol: one of 20 and 4 of 10 injections each. The wound is entirely healed and there is no evidence on palpation of any recurrence on examination to-day. (Nov. 16th, 1936). Patient is working, has gained weight and looks and feels in excellent health.

K.A., age 32 Struck dorsum of right foot on piece of iron, March, 1933. One month later small tumor-like growth appeared and 5 mos. later had increased in size and was excised and a diagnosis of spindle-cell sarcoma made. Had extensive X-ray and radium treatment. Six months later, nodules appeared in right groin and a little later in the right popliteal space which soon enlarged to the size of an apple. Had proliferative, ulcerating mass on dorsum of foot. Began Ensol treatment Nov. 20, 1935, and showed a very definite pain reaction when dosage reached certain amounts, this reaction being centred in the tumor masses. These tumor masses gradually became softer and finally semi-fluctuant. The mass on the dorsum of the foot showed extensive slough and there occurred at one time a fairly brisk venous hemorrhage from this site. Had one course of 20 and one of 10 injections of Ensol and about one week after completion of 2nd course the whole inguinal mass sloughed away and there was considerable sloughing of the mass on the dorsum of the foot. Patient, however, continued to regress and died about ten days following this and approximately 5 mos. after beginning the Ensol treatment.

There appeared in this case to be a very definite reaction in the tumor tissue to the Ensol injections and with none of the other types of treatment, radium, X-ray, etc., did he experience the reaction and changes that occurred with it.

Mrs. K., age 43 yrs. Menorrhagia and metrorrhagia for 2 yrs. with a loss of 22 lbs. in the past 7 mos. Examination shows marked narrowing of the upper half of the vagina, the cervix being high on the left side. The body of the uterus is not defined but apparently included in a mass the size of a 2 1/2 mos. pregnancy and lying more to the right. The mass is hard, smooth and fairly movable. Panhysterectomy was performed and an extensive adenocarcinoma of the body of the uterus was found markedly infiltrating the uterine walls. Had one course of deep X-ray therapy and 2 mos. after this began Ensol treatment on Jan.

17th, 1936. Has had 5 courses of Ensol, one of 20 injections and 4 of 10 injections each. Has gained weight, looks and feels well, is stronger and as far as examination, at the present time, shows, there is no evidence of recurrence.

J.W.M., male, age 65 years Difficulty in swallowing for two months. Has lost 40 lbs. in 5 months. No solid food for two months. X-ray examination reveals a carcinoma of the oesophagus at the mid-sternal level. Refused gastrostomy. Began Ensol treatment Dec. 24, 1935. Did not show any particular immediate benefit although he felt that there was probably slightly less difficulty in swallowing. On completion of 20 injections he left for his home on the prairie. About ten weeks after his return home, he noticed very definitely less dysphagia, began to put on weight and gained in strength to such an extent that he was able to act as census-taker and was quite active in his duties. Had 3 other courses of Ensol at home, given by his family doctor, and for some months felt quite comfortable, but gradually began to fail and died 10 mos. after beginning treatment.

Mrs. B., age 75 25 yrs. ago, she bumped leg against a stool and ruptured a vein; since then there has existed a more or less non-healing ulcer. 6 mos. ago, fell from chair, striking the same leg and aggravating the old injury, the ulceration spreading, edges heaping up and becoming foul. Has lost some weight. Local examination shows in the skin of the right anterior tibial region, an extensive ulcerating carcinomatous appearing growth 22 x 12 cms. with proliferating, papillary edges and bleeding readily on touching. Inguinal glands are enlarged and from biopsy of growth, Oct. 2nd, 1935, it shows a squamous-cell carcinoma, grade 2. X-ray of leg, Oct. 9th shows "extensive infiltration of greater part of middle third of right tibia, especially anterior half, with a neoplastic growth, probably direct invasion. There is extensive periostitis involving the attachment of the interosseous membrane both tibia and fibula." She began Ensol treatment Oct. 15th, 1935, and had 17 injections between this time and Nov. 27th, when she refused further treatment. No particular change was noted in the growth, except that it appeared cleaner and seemed to be granulating slightly at margins. She was transferred to a convalescent annex where she died Dec. 20th, 1935, and at autopsy showed the ulcerated growth to measure only 15 x 8 cms. and the inguinal glands not involved. There was an extensive osteomyelitis of the right tibia, chronic nephritis, sclerotic, mitral and aortic endocarditis. Sections through the growth on leg showed extensive vacuolation and swelling of the nuclei of the carcinomatous cells, which we have noted in other sections from Ensol-treated cases.

S.D.,male, age 35 yrs. Epigastric discomfort after meals and gradual loss of weight for the past 6 yrs. Epigastric soreness past 5-6 months. In 1929 these symptoms began and the soreness developed during the summer of 1935; occasional vomiting; X-ray diagnosis of carcinoma of pyloric end of stomach made and on Aug. 4th, 1935, had pyloric resection performed. Sometime after operation, began to vomit. Was home for a while and then readmitted to hospital and continuous gastric suction and intravenous glucose-saline used. Very emaciated but no definite masses palpable and X-ray of stomach taken Oct. 18th, 1935, shows barium meal still present in the stomach at end of 5 hrs. Began Ensol treatment Oct. 2nd, 1935, and in about 2 weeks began to take liquids by mouth with very little discomfort and X-ray on Nov. 8th, 1935, showed stomach to be empty at end of 5 hrs. and no definite evidence of organic lesion. Stoma functioning well. In 2 months, had gained 15 lbs., was eating solids without discomfort, driving own car. Between date of discharge from hospital, Nov. 10th, and Mar. 30th, 1936, when he returned for 3rd course of Ensol, he had been steadily gaining weight (approximately 30 lbs.) and strength, was working daily and feeling well except for occasional "sour stomach" and vomiting. Early in April he began to feel much weaker, considerable gastric and epigastric distress, loss of weight and appetite and regressed fairly steadily till his death, May 15th, 1936. There was quite remarkable improvement in this patient for some months, and whether the obstruction of the stoma was neoplastic or inflammatory, it is difficult to say, and if the seeming benefit from the beginning of Ensol therapy, was merely coincidental.

BULLETIN

OF THE

HENDRY-CONNELL
RESEARCH FOUNDATION

NO. 3

CANCER RESEARCH

MARCH, 1938

KINGSTON, ONT. CANADA

CONTENTS OF BULLETIN NO. 3 *

ENSOL AT WILMINGTON
Case Histories
G.A.C., MD

The following case histories are reported from the Wilmington Cancer Research Foundation of which Dr. G.A.C. is Director and Dr. J.M.B. is Consultant. The Ensol used was supplied partly from the Kingston laboratory and partly from the laboratory of the Biochemical Research Foundation of the Franklin Institute at Philadelphia.

Case 1 Mr. C.H. In November, 1934, the patient had a pain in RLQ which became progressively worse. He was treated for intestinal grippe and this treatment did not help the patient. The pain got worse, patient lost his appetite, lost weight and strength. He complained that his stomach would swell and would only be relieved by considerable belching. In February, 1935, an operation was performed during which part of the cecum was resected and an end to side anastomosis performed. The resected gut contained a mass which was later diagnosed as scirrhous carcinoma. Shortly after the operation the pain returned to the RLQ and has remained up to the time Ensol was started. The patient still complained of loss of weight and strength. The patient was

*All these articles are available on request. See appendix.

59

still complained of loss of weight and strength. The patient was referred to me on August 14, 1936, an X-ray was made at this time which showed an irregular defect involving lower two-thirds of caecum. It was extremely tender and fixed. Ensol was started on August 17th. One-half hour after each injection of 1 cc the patient experiences a "pins and needles" sensation and a pulling feeling in RLQ. At present the dose is 1 cc daily without a rest period.

Today the patient has no pain and has no tenderness in his RLQ. He has gained three pounds and is capable of working a whole day in the fields, cutting corn, etc. The patient says that he now feels like two men.

Conclusion Appetite has improved-No pain in RLQ even on deep palpation. Gain in weight and is capable of doing a day's work without suffering any ill effects. All his previous signs and symptoms of cancer have disappeared.

Dec. 10th, 1936. During the past month there has been very little change. He has, however, gained two more pounds and has no symptoms whatsoever. I had him X-rayed on August 17th, 1936, before starting treatment. The following is the report:

Barium enema progressed without delay or distress to the caecum. The descending and transverse colon mass freely movable and not tender. No filling defects or areas of spasm seen. The caecum shows a constant irregular defect involving its entire lower 2/3. It was extremely tender and partially fixed. After elimination the colon appears normal except for the defect in the caecum. Barium meal shows the same defect without residue in the ileum at ten hours.

Conclusion Recurrent carcinoma of the caecum, without obstruction. (See photograph of the film.)

After three months' treatment I again had him X-rayed and the report is as follows:

The barium enema progressed very rapidly and without distress to the caecum. The descending colon and the distal half of the transverse was smooth-walled-freely movable and not tender. No filling defects or areas of spasm noted. The ascending colon and the proximal half of transverse colon showed widely spaced shallow haustral markings. The caecum was not completely filled at any

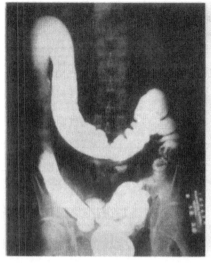
Fig. 1. Case 1 – First X-ray

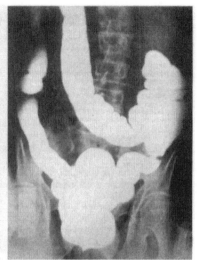
Fig. 2. Case 1 – Second X-ray

time, but was freely movable and not tender. The radiographs show a constant defect of the caecum. The lumen, however, is larger and the walls appear somewhat smoother than at the examination of 8-18-36. The examination, four hours after barium meal, shows about one-half the barium still in the terminal ileum. Caecum shows the same defect as shown in the barium enema. The six hour study shows the ileum practically empty.

Conclusion There is a constant defect in the caecum with no evidence of obstruction. Comparison with the examination of 8-18-36 shows considerable improvement. (See photograph of the film.)

I was certainly amazed to see the marked improvement and the decrease in the size of the mass.

Dec. 17th, 1936. Continues quite well.

Case 2 *Mrs. S.W.* Three years ago the patient was operated upon and a mass was found on the lesser curvature of the stomach which by biopsy was diagnosed as adeno-carcinoma. Patient has been taking morph. sulph. and pantopon at different times to control pain. Physical examination shows a markedly emaciated female practically bed-ridden. Her liver is on a level with the umbilicus. In the epigastrium there is a hard mass about the size of a grapefruit which is fixed. She has considerable ascites. Injections with Ensol were commenced on

September 9th, 1936. One-half hour after each injection the patient complains of a pulling sensation and "pins and needles" sensation in area of cancer. Her pain has been definitely checked and she does not require any opiates.

Dec. 10th, 1936. This patient I treated for two and one-half months and definitely stopped her pain. She had the usual sensations following 1cc doses of No. 47. She died two weeks ago and I was given permission to obtain a piece of the cancer. I used a new blade in cutting this tissue and I might say that it was with great difficulty that I was able to cut a piece from the growth. Grossly it showed considerable fibrosis. I am waiting for a microscopical report from Dr. McDonald.

Case 3 Mrs. E.M., age 57 yrs. In August, 1935, patient complained of vaginal bleeding. This increased until she consulted a physician who advised biopsy of cervix. Upon examining the cervix it was found that the entire cervix had eroded away leaving a crater. Biopsy showed undifferentiated cancer tissue. Patient lost 28 pounds up to September 23rd of this year. She lost strength steadily and during August was confined to bed with pain and weakness. In August, 1936, she was sent to the hospital and received deep X-ray. Following this she returned home and was still confined to her bed with pain and weakness. Injections with Ensol were started on September 23rd, 1 cc per day being the dose given. Today the patient has an excellent appetite and is able to do work around the house and go to town. She has no pain and no vaginal discharge. She now weighs 196 pounds, a gain of 22 pounds since September 23rd.

Dec. 10th, 1936. She has no symptoms of cancer at present and is able to walk around without any difficulty. In my last report she weighed 196 pounds, a gain of 22 pounds since treatment started September 23rd. Today she weighs 202 pounds or a gain of 28 pounds. Dose of 1 cc daily of No. 47.

Dec. 17th, 1936. Last report. Continues quite well.

Case 4 Female. Age 37. For the past four months the patient complained of progressive weakness and loss of weight. She had a steady pain in RLQ. In July she noticed her abdomen swelling and this swelling became progressive until she was operated on August 26th, 1936. A large right ovarian cyst was removed and diagnosed as adenocarcinoma (very malignant and rapid-spreading). Ensol treatment was commenced on September 28th, the dose being 1 cc per day. To date her appetite has improved, she has no pain, is out and around, and has gained four pounds.

Dec. 10th, 1936. This patient has a good appetite. Slight pain at times in cancer area. During good weather she walks to my office, a distance of a mile, for treatment without much effort. Since my last report she has gained two more pounds, making a total gain of six pounds since September 28th. She has been getting 1.5 cc's of No. 47 daily.

Dec. 17th, 1936. No signs or symptoms of cancer. Appears to be as well as before the onset of malignancy.

Case 5 Male. Age 54. In August, 1936, patient's right chest was opened at Johns Hopkins Hospital. A large bronchiogenic cancer of upper and middle lobe of right lung, with metastasis to mediastinum was found. Patient was immediately closed and later sent home. Ensol injections were started on September 28th, the dose being 1 cc per day. After each injection the patient said he had a pulling feeling in the right chest. After fourteen injections the old incision in the right chest opened and about a quart of odorless pinkish purulent material drained out. Mixed in with this pinkish purulent material was a large amount of necrotic tissue. Patient's pain had disappeared and his appetite was the best in months. Culture of his exudates show gram-negative bacilli. The USPH also isolated a subspecies of salmonella morgani, castellani and chalmers. One week later, after receiving 30 cc of blood during a transfusion the patient went into shock and died. His right lung was removed and upon section purulent material exuded from meshes of fibrous tissue. The majority of lung had liquified.

A report of lung section is as follows: The lung showed on section an adenocarcinoma with the lung tissue itself obliterated completely, either replaced or so necrotic that it is not recognized. A culture of tissue in veal broth showed several types of organisms or several forms of the same one.

Case 6 Cambridge. Age 63. Diagnosed as adenocarcinoma of ovary. Cancer metastasis to right lung. Ensol treatments commenced on October 1st. Her doctor wrote me that after two weeks treatment her general condition has improved and that she has less pain. She sleeps well and takes nourishment fairly well.

Dec. 10th, 1936. This patient feels much better. She has very little pain and her appetite has improved. She was able to go out of the house the first time in months and is up and around each day. Her doctor is very much satisfied with her condition.

Dec. 17th, 1936. Last report. Continues to improve.

Case 7 Male. Age 65. By X-ray and clinical diagnosis a malignancy of lower colon was made. An operation was performed and the tumor and colon were transfixed outside the abdomen prior to the second state of resection. The blood supply was left intact. 10 cc of Ensol was injected into the mass, and after four days it was removed. Grossly it showed beginning necrosis of mass.

Dec. 10th, 1936. A section showed principally fatty reticulum with some large supporting septa. One section showed considerable blood pigment. However, there is no evidence of any malignancy.

Dr. T.P., a Boston orthopedic surgeon, has been using Ensol on two patients. The following is an extract of a letter which I have just received from him:

> I have now used Ensol on two patients – the first patient refused treatment after the first dose; the second patient was a woman who had a lipomyxosarcoma with metastasis to the brain cubital spaces, and she had an amputation by me in September. The diagnosis of this tumor was made by three different men.
>
> At the time I started giving her Ensol she was receiving 1/2gr of morphine every three hours for twenty-four hours. I gave her the treatment every other day and every third day. After the first dose of 1 cc I noted a marked difference of morphine taken. I took the opportunity to inject into the tumor in the left cubital space one-half the dose and noted there was a very decided softening in the tumor immediately and a decrease in size of the tumor.

A case from Toronto W.R.–Age 40 years. In August, 1933, patient passed a few drops of blood after urination.

In October, 1934, had quite a large haemorrhage, and one hour later passed clots. One month later had another large haemorrhage. A cystoscopy was performed by a good man, and a complete resection of the bladder advised due to the large size of the growth. He had been given arsenical treatment for his lues without improvement.

Functional Inquiry This was essentially negative except for a chronic cough.

Physical Examination Colour looked fair-abdomen slightly tender above the pubes.

Reflexes normal.

Cervical axillary inguinal glands enlarged II+.

Per rectum-the prostate was small, and the bladder could be felt fixed to the rectum.

Laboratory Findings *Urine:* Alkaline, albumin II+, sugar negative, red blood cells III+, pus II+.

Blood: Haemoglobin 98%, erythrocytes 4,880,000, leucocytes 6600, Wasserman Kolman IV+, Kahn III+.

X-ray Findings *Chest:* Fibrosis of both lungs.

Pelvic Bones: Negative for metastases.

Cystogram The cystogram shows a large filling defect in the bladder.

Diagnosis Carcinoma of the bladder.

It was felt that there was too much fixation to the rectal wall to allow successful resection, and as the patient had not improved under anti-luetic treatment, he should be given a course of selenium treatment with deep X-ray therapy.

This procedure was carried out, but cystogram about four months later showed no appreciable reduction in the size of the tumour, and no improvement in the haematuria.

On several occasions during the course of treatment by deep X-ray it was necessary to wash the bladder free of clots to ease his suffering. We felt that the patient was making little progress, and as a last resort he was sent to Kingston for treatment with Ensol.

He reported back to Toronto during his course in Kingston with considerable improvement in symptoms and some gain in weight. Following a continuance of treatment with Ensol his haematuria disappeared.

I was called out to see him one night, and secured the following history:

He had been feeling very well, and there had been no haematuria. After finishing a course of Ensol he had decided to visit friends in the country, and after taking a laxative one cold night found it necessary to make several trips to an outdoor privy. A chill followed and he came on to Toronto. He complained of marked frequency, dysuria, and pain over both kidney cells. A diagnosis of pyelonephritis was made, and he was brought into hospital. The patient did not improve under treatment, but became progressively more toxic and died.

Permission could be obtained for only a limited post mortem. The abdomen was apparently free of metastases. Both kidneys showed a marked degree of pyelonephritis. On opening the bladder, we were amazed at the apparent disappearance of the tumour. The mucous membrane of the bladder was much whiter than normal. The trigone and prostatic area felt very rubbery to the touch. The bladder was excised, and a portion of the trigonal area sent for section.

Microscopic Report This tissue consists almost entirely of a malignant tumour growth composed of atypical epithelial cells of the transitional type. Practically no normal mucosa is present, the mucosal surface showed very marked degeneration. Throughout the muscle coat tumour cells are found invading between the muscle bundles separating them rather widely from their neighbours. These cells varied quite markedly in size, shape, and staining characters, and a number of mitotic figures are present.

Diagnosis Transitional cell carcinoma of the bladder.

This patient was admitted to the Kingston Clinic, Oct. 22, 1935.

Note in report We felt that the patient was making little progress, and as a last resort he was sent to Kingston for treatment with Ensol. He reported back to Toronto during his course in Kingston with considerable improvement in symptoms and some gain in weight. Following a continuance of treatment with Ensol his haematuria disappeared.

Ensol was used from Oct. 22nd to Nov. 25th, 1935, when he was given a rest period. On the day following his first treatment the burning pain was greatly eased. Oct. 30th, passed by urethra considerable quantity of fleshy material. Nov. 8th, general improvement, less pain, gain in weight of 5 1/2 lbs. Nov. 30th, no haematuria, less frequent urination. Home.

Comment As in so many other cases Ensol was "a last resort" and, as in some others, not all, there was a definite result. For confirmation of the result see post mortem report, "On opening the bladder, we were amazed at the apparent disappearance of the tumor."

CASE HISTORIES, KINGSTON CLINIC

C.D.T. MUNDELL, BA, MD
I. SUTTON, MD
G.S. BURTON, MD
W.A. CAMPBELL, MD

Case histories in this bulletin are in categories. In Bulletin No. 1 an effort was made to classify cases on a basis of results. This proved to be difficult and unsatisfactory, partly because of the interim character of the reports and further because of difference of opinion in determining the nature and value of results. The present classification is exact for it is based upon the status of the case when taken on for treatment. Each reader can form his own estimate of the result in each case. The categories used are as follows:

1. Cases diagnosed malignant which refused surgery and/or radiation.
2. Early cases which had surgery and/or radiation, the use of Ensol being added in the hope of assisting in prevention of extension or recurrence.
3. Cases diagnosed malignant, clinically or by biopsy, pronounced inoperable and not suitable for radiation and regarded as hopeless.
4. Cases upon which all the resources of surgery and radiation had been employed and then pronounced incurable and hopeless.

Category 1

Cases which were suitable for other treatment but refused it

Case 34 *An early case which refused operation or radiation. Mrs. F.M.C., age 62. Malignant papilloma, rectum.*

July 17th, 1935, patient writes "A week ago Dr. ... told me he had discovered that I had cancer of the rectum. The only thing, he said, to do was to operate and remove the growth, that would mean removing the rectum, as well as making an artificial opening in the lower side of the abdomen, I would rather die than have this done." Biopsy report, July 8th, 1935, "From the general character of the cells, their arrangement, their variation in size and deep staining properties, we believe this to be probably malignant." The early symptoms were digestive disturbance, abdominal pain, loss of weight, irregular diarrhoea with traces of blood. Admitted Aug. 1st, 1935. Treated with Ensol to Aug.

28th. There were seventeen treatments of about 13 cc's in all. There was a rapid recovery, appetite improved, general condition better, weight increased, stools became well formed and painless. Sept. 27th, another biopsy examination. Doubt expressed as to the malignant nature of the cells to be seen in slides. Nov. 26th, 1935, in good health, has resumed her usual life. Dec. 10th, 1935, no evidence of recurrence. All symptoms have disappeared. Gain of 20 lbs. in weight. June 10th, 1936, no evidence of recurrence. Oct. 8th, 1936, continues well.

Rectal examination report The anterior wall which was involved in the original examination is clear on palpation. High up in the ampulla a fold can be made out. This is on the left lateral wall. It is not nodular but gives the sensation of being thickened. Using the short proctoscope there is no constriction of the lumen at this level. The thickened area does not bleed and is not inflamed. It is at a level approximately 10 cms from the anus.

Blood examination Routine blood examination showed RBC 5, 030,000, Hgb. 103. Regular blood chemistry normal. Fasting blood sugar 113.

Comment The rapid and complete recovery in this case and continued good health after fifteen months, has placed the original diagnosis in doubt. However, there was loss of health and a mass in the rectum. If it were benign it disappeared while Ensol was being administered and shortly thereafter, and all symptoms with it. Even this is unusual and remarkable.

Case 62 *Mrs. J.G.I., age 40. Carcinoma, rectum.*
Biopsy proof. First symptom March, 1935, periodic bleeding from rectum, some diarrhoea and tenesmus (involuntary straining). Colostomy advised but refused. Examination showed a mass on the anterior wall with a sloughing ulcer completing the circle of the rectum. Aug. 6th, 1935, Ensol treatments begun, patient showed immediate local and general improvement. Nov. 15th, Dr. M. writes "Patient feels practically free from all symptoms. Ulceration has had a tendency each time to dry up after treatment but not quite so marked this last period." March 4th, 1936, "Growth unchanged for the past two months" May 16th, 1936, the rectal mass is very bulky with great fringe of papilliferous edges. Ulcerated area not sore and does not bleed, abdomen clear. Aug. 28th, 1936, fairly comfortable, no pain, bowels regular,

some discharge, appetite good but no gain in weight. Sept. 11th, 1936, the mass is now involving the posterior vaginal wall. General condition remains the same. Sept. 26th, 1936, remains remarkably comfortable even though the growth is extending. Treated at home.

Case 674 Mrs. L.C., age 66. Carcinoma, breast, right.
Clinical diagnosis. First symptom two years ago, had cracked nipple, then tumor formed under nipple which became retracted. Ulceration followed and slowly increased. No treatment. Refused surgery or radiation. Ensol used April 29th, 1936, to date. Under treatment ulcer became much cleaner but the mass did not change in size. Oct. 12th, 1936, one soft axillary gland palpable, seems to be inflammatory rather than malignant. Nov. 16th, 1936, gland no longer palpable, mass and ulceration unchanged.

Case 685 Mrs. I.S., age 67. Rodent ulcer, temporal angle of jaw.
Biopsy proof. Extension subcutaneously behind jaw. Ensol used May 17th to Sept. 5th., when she went home feeling very well, good appetite, weight increased from 123 to 129 lbs. June 5th, the ridge from ear to scar is definitely softer. Sept. 4th, subcutaneous area behind ear has disappeared, anterior crusted nodule dryer. No later report.

Category 2

Cases treated for prevention of extension or recurrence

Case 101 Mrs. A. McC., age 69. Carcinoma, breast, right.
Biopsy proof. First symptom Sept., 1934, noticed tumor which was removed. Ensol used from Aug. 19th to Nov. 6th, general improvement, felt well, appetite good, little pain. No report later.

Case 144 Surgery with Enso*l* – *Mrs. G.I., age 46.* Carcinoma, right breast.
Biopsy proof. First symptoms late in 1934, noted tumor in right breast, later bloody discharge from nipple, aching pain. Admitted Aug. 22nd, 1935. Operation, mastectomy, then treated with Ensol, continued at intervals up to the present. Jan. 10th, 1936, incision healed, some keloid, no glands palpable. May 8th, no evidence of recurrence. July 10th, no evidence of recurrence. Sept. 18th, continues well.

Case 271 Mrs. H.W.L., age 42. Carcinoma, breast.
Biopsy proof. First symptoms March, 1935, noticed small painless tumor, later removed with the breast, April 30th, 1935. Admitted Oct. 4th, 1935, for preventive treatment. First Ensol Oct. 4th, treatment continued to Nov. 8th. Second course Feb. 21st to 29th, feels well. Third course June 9th to 13th, in good condition. Sept. 2nd to 9th, very well, increased in weight from 134 to 144 1/2 lbs., no evidence of spread, X-ray clear.

Case 362 Mrs. J.R., age 58. Carcinoma, right ovary.
Biopsy proof. Operation, partial resection Nov. 20th, 1934. Menopause six years ago. Developed pain in right side of abdomen in Feb. 1934. Admitted Oct. 22nd, 1935, abdomen not distended, no palpable masses, slight tenderness in lower quadrant, right, no evidence of recurrence in the wall. No bowel obstruction. Treated Oct. 22nd, 1935, to Oct. 1936. General condition remained good. Jan. 3rd, 1936, nothing palpable in abdomen. Feb. 21st, condition unchanged. April 3rd, same. June 5th, very well. Sept. 5th, treatment continued. Oct. 4th, 1936, not so well.

Case 448 L. McK., age 34. Carcinoma, testicle.
Biopsy proof. First symptom Aug., 1935, swelling of right testicle, progressively larger, firm and painless. Operation in Oct., followed by good recovery. Biopsy to make diagnosis. Ensol used, postoperative to prevent recurrence, Nov. 22nd, 1935, to March 28th, 1936. Jan. 16th, 1936, no evidence of recurrence or metastases. March 27th, 1936, still clear.

Case 788 J.B.A.P., age 34. Carcinoma, testicle, left.
Biopsy. Orchidectomy Aug. 15th, 1936. First symptom six years ago. Swelling in the body of the testis, increased slowly till Nov., 1935, when there was marked enlargement which subsided in March, 1936. Increased again, Operation Aug., 1936. Deep X-ray, four treatments post-operative to lumbar and lumbo-sacral regions. On admission, Sept. 14th, 1936, complained of weakness in the back in lumbar region, dull ache if lying or sitting long in one position, loss of appetite. Scar of incision in groin well healed, thickening not excessive, no mass palpable in left groin. Is luetic. Ensol used Sept. 16th to

Oct. 24th, 1936, pain in back disappeared. Oct. 18th, no complaints, fairly comfortable. Oct. 24th, 1936. Home.

Category 3

Cases pronounced inoperable and hopeless,
not suitable for other treatment

Case 20 *J.B., age 76.* Carcinoma, stomach.
Clinical diagnosis. First symptom, poor health for five or six years. Decline rapid in past five months. Blockage in stomach confirmed by X-ray. Admitted July 26th, 1935, treated with Ensol to Sept. 1st, with very marked improvement, appetite returned, took regular meals, gained in weight. Discharged to report to outpatient department but did not do so. Died, March 29th, 1936.

Case 64 *N.S., age 65.* Carcinoma, rectum.
Clinical proof only. Aug. 5th, 1935, admitted for treatment, complained of general weakness, intermittent pain across lower abdomen and in rectum, alternating periods of diarrhoea and constipation. Duration of condition approximately ten months. First Ensol treatment Aug. 6th, treated for one month. Gained in weight from 129 to 140 lbs., less discomfort and large stools noted during treatment. No further Ensol treatment. March 20th, 1936, Dr. L. writes "Patient is suffering from partial obstruction. The lower end of the growth has lessened but apparently increased higher up. In spite of condition he has returned to work."

Case 88 *Mrs. A.G., age 62.* Carcinoma, rectum.
Clinical diagnosis, later biopsy. First symptom Oct. 34th, pain in rectum, worse when sitting, bleeding, increasing constipation, pain in left hip. Ensol used Aug. 13th to Dec. 22nd, 1935. Sept. 14th, general condition improved, pain variable. Nov. 6th, 1935, letter, Dr. S., freer from pain, generally better, weight stationary, mass in rectum smaller.

Case 161 *Mrs. L.S., age 57.* Carcinoma, breast.
Biopsy proof. First symptom 1934. This was a mental case at Ontario Hospital. There were hard nodules in the breast with secondaries in the axillary glands. Ensol was first used Sept. 6th, 1935. By Oct. 21st she was mentally well and returned to Toronto to have the breast removed.

Feb. 16th, 1936, reported at clinic quite well. April 25th, 1936, feels fine. July 27th, 1936, quite well.

Comment Patient's mental diagnosis was a depressive condition precipitated by worry over her malignancy. Under Ensol treatment she improved physically and as anxiety lessened, the depressive symptoms gradually cleared up, and she returned to her former good health. Since operation she has remained quite well.

Case 249 J. McL., age 50. Carcinoma glands, right side of neck.
Biopsy. First symptoms early in 1935, notice small painless tumor on right side of neck which gradually enlarged up to Sept. when biopsy was done and diagnosis made of basal cell ca. Ensol used Sept. 28th to Oct. 25th, 1935. Improved, then home to be treated with Ensol there. Dr. S. reported in May, 1936, marked improvement in weight and health generally. Examined in Kingston clinic on May 5th, 1936, general condition good, still gaining in weight, appetite good and sleeps well, no pain. X-ray negative for secondaries. Returned to Dr. S. for continued treatment.

Case 255 X-ray combined with Ensol – *F.S., age 40.* Carcinoma, nasal bones and ethmoidal cells.
Biopsy proof. First symptoms May, 1935, frontal headache, pain over bridge of nose with tenderness, slight swelling: then all symptoms increased, both sides of nose involved, then discharge. Operation followed. Dr. M. writes, "We had considerable difficulty in reaching a diagnosis as tissue removed on several occasions showed only inflammatory growth. Finally, however, wider exploration was carried out and firm tissue found which proved, on section, to be squamous celled carcinoma." Radiologist at St. Michael's Hospital thought the case not suitable for radiation therapy and sent him for Ensol. First treated with Ensol Oct. 1st, 1935. X-ray report, Oct. 1st. "... the nasal bone has completely disappeared, and the lower central portion of the frontal bone has also been destroyed. The frontal process of the maxillary bone has also been destroyed, and both maxillary antra are hazy." Oct. 3rd, had deep X-ray. Oct. 19th, feels fine, no pain. Oct. 23rd, very well (see photographs). Jan. 18th, 1936, home, well. April 14th, 1936, no evidence of recurrence. Second X-ray report, Nov. 20th, 1935: "... accessory nasal sinuses present an appearance quite similar to that seen

before except that at this time some of the haziness due to soft tissue formation in the region of the destroyed bone has disappeared. The antra are still hazy but are practically the same as in the previous films." Third X-ray report, Jan. 14th, 1936: "The frontal sinuses are clearer than in the previous films. The right antrum has always been quite clear. The left antrum is now less hazy than previously. The bony erosion of the nasal and frontal bones previously noted is still present but there has been some clearing of the congestion of the sinuses, particularly on the left side."

Comment This, it will be noted was a case of combined Ensol and deep X-ray treatment. As in other similar cases the radiologist has stated that the improvement was due to radiation alone. While that may be the case, Ensol is not to be disposed of so easily. An unbiased, open-minded radiologist with some aptitude for research is needed who will combine Ensol with radiation in a series of cases to learn what impression it makes upon them, both those which respond readily to radiation and those which are refractory or resistant.

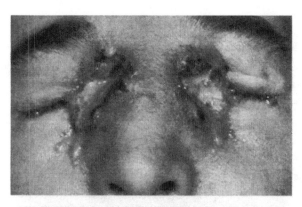

Fig. 5
Case 255, F.S.

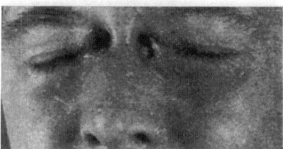

Fig. 6
Case 255, F.S.
Two months later

Case 311 H.J.M., age 62. Carcinoma, stomach.

Diagnosis by X-ray. First symptoms summer of 1934. Complains of easy fatigue, food stays in stomach, vomiting, gas forms, cramping pains in legs and feet, constipated. First treated with Ensol Oct. 16th, 1935, improved slowly. Nov. 6th, feels fairly well. Dec. 6th, condition unchanged. Feb. 8th, 1936, feels very well. March 28th, not much change. June 12th, nothing palpable over the epigastric region. July 19th, home, feeling very well. Home with Ensol. Sept. 28th, reported back in fair condition, weight maintained, working. Oct. 23rd, 1936, no mass palpable in epigastrium, general condition fairly good, has been working all summer. Home again with Ensol.

Case 446 Mrs. L.F., age 67. Carcinoma, vulva, epidermoid.

Biopsy proof. First symptoms Aug., 1935, noted she had to urinate frequently, accompanied with burning and itching. Rubbing produced abrasion of skin that would not heal. Urinary symptoms increased in severity. First treated with Ensol Jan. 17th, 1936, combined with X-ray. Continued to Feb. 21st. March 18th, writes, "Am writing to let you know I am healed and feeling fine, don't think I shall have to come back for treatment."

Case 519 E.R.L., age 64. Carcinoma, rectum.

Biopsy proof. First symptoms, Sept., 1935, heavy feeling in rectum, frequent defecation, gas in bowels, pain down left leg. Admitted Dec. 27th, 1935. Ensol used here and in Utica since with rest periods. In the first courses there was some improvement in the local condition. In March and April pain increased and ulcer became larger. In June there was pain control and advance seemed checked. Aug. 14th, 1936, pain controlled, growth less in size, less tenderness and no spasm, general condition good. Oct. 12th, 1936, little tenderness or spasm, ulcer does not bleed, general condition holding. Nov. 19th, 1936, pain returned with increasing bowel difficulty. Home with Ensol to Dr. M.

Case 775 Mrs. G.B.W., age 38. Carcinoma, primary lesion uncertain, secondaries in axilla and X-ray after admission showed extensive bone involvement.

Vaginal examination found cervix has a transverse bilateral tear, thick yellowish discharge, surface eroded, bleeds on palpation, edge not friable. On admission, Sept. 2nd, 1936, complained of weakness and stiffness in right leg, groin and back, shooting pains through hips, general weakness, appetite fair. Ensol used Sept. 3rd to 16th. As she was failing rapidly was advised to go home. Left Sept. 16th in poor condition. Oct. 5th, 1936, telegram from Dr. C. stated remarkable change for the better. Ensol sent for home use.

Comment Ensol was used for 13 days only, before she was sent home in a hopeless condition. Yet it is noted that the effects of even that short period of treatment became so marked that there was a hurried call for Ensol to be used at home.

Category 4
Cases upon which all the resources of surgery and radiation had been employed and then pronounced incurable and hopeless

Case 3 M.J.V., age 40. Carcinoma, stomach, obstruction of pylorus. July, 1934. Symptoms began with a dull gnawing pain in the epigastrium. This was accentuated by spiced foods or fried meats. At first it was apparent only after meals and was relieved by evicting gas. Later it gradually lengthened until he was always conscious of a sense of weight there, which flared into definite burning pain. Appetite began to fail in September, 1934. Previous to this he "could eat anything." Then he developed a distaste for potatoes and was not interested in his meals. He was examined by X-ray in Don Jail, Toronto, in September, 1935, and a diagnosis of duodenal ulcer made. He was placed on a modified sippy diet. Further examination in the Kingston General Hospital showed a constant filling deformity at the pylorus and a partial twenty-four-hour retention. Diagnosis of carcinoma of the stomach was made. April 12th, 1935. Complaints: 1. Pain, constant and burning in character, in the pit of the stomach, at times referred to the liver area, to the heart and to the spine. 2. Loss of appetite, specific for greasy foods, milk, potatoes, spices, poor for all foods and small quantities fill him up. 3. Loss of weight estimated at 50 lbs. in the past eight months. 4. Vomiting, persistent till recently, after meals, gave no relief, at times dark and tarry. 5. Constipation marked. In appearance is a well-developed but moderately wasted man, colour grey, lips and surfaces pale, general appearance sullen but face is drawn as in dyspeptics, wasting marked in hands and legs, abdomen still has subcutaneous fat, tongue heavily coated and breath offensive. Operation, May 31st, 1935. A scirrhus growth at the pylorus involving 3 1/2" showing early peritoneal involvement. Glands along lesser curvature and at celiac axis. Posterior gastro-enterostomy was done. This man was serving a term in the Kingston Penitentiary and was granted a pardon upon the report of the surgeon following this operation. He was referred for treatment with Ensol on June 14th, 1935. June 15th, first Ensol used, continued daily. June 21st, appetite good, eating all foods except fried meats. No distaste for any foods. Gained 1 1/2 lbs. in weight. July 2nd, 1935, X-ray report: "Only the fundus of the stomach is seen, the pylorus being completely obliterated. The barium is seen leaving the stomach through the gastro-enterostomy opening. July 9th, gained 3 lbs. in weight in seven days. July 7th, discharged from hospital to Outpatient Dept. Patient feels better than at any time since illness began. July 17th, given permission to go to Montreal on business. July 30th, returned feeling very fit, appetite good, eats everything, gained 6 lbs. in weight while away. Treatment resumed." Aug. 10th, 1935, X-ray report "No particular difference in the area of the shadow of that part of the fundus of the stomach which is filled with barium. However, it was possible to manipulate the stomach in such a way in the screening that the pylorus was filled in part, and some of the barium spilled out through the duodenum." From Sept. 1935, to Jan. 12th, 1936, he remained in Montreal apparently in good health. Weight remained at 170 lbs., a gain of 2 1/2 lbs. since the beginning of treatment. When he returned in January, he was feeling not quite so well. As he had been going about Montreal apparently quite fit, it was proposed to return him to the Kingston Penitentiary to complete his sentence. However, apart from worry over this prospect he was not so well, but he was unwilling to remain long in Kingston for treatment. He was treated for short periods in March, April, June and July and felt better but did not return to former good condition, and he again lost in weight. After a month's absence he returned with persistent vomiting, becoming weaker. Finally he refused further treatment, went to Montreal where he died Sept. 25th, 1936. X-ray report of Aug. 21st, 1936, stated that there was progression of the disease.

Comment Soon after operation and the beginning of treatment with Ensol this man recovered normal health and retained it for about a year. Then relapse and fatal termination in about two months. Unfortunately a post mortem could not be secured. Did surgery give him the extra year of life? Did Ensol play a part in the temporary recovery?

Case 26 Mrs. R.B.S., age 42. Carcinoma, left breast, scirrhous, with widespread secondaries.

Biopsy proof. See original report, Bulletin No. 1, page 20. "The pelvic girdle and lower lumbar vertebrae were involved, and there was a pathological fracture of the hip. Treatment with Ensol was commenced on July 27th. By Aug. 14th pain was well controlled, and extension was applied to straighten the left leg. On Aug. 19th X-ray examination showed that there was no evidence of further involvement." First symptoms were in 1932. Mastectomy in Aug. 1933. Sept. 9th and Nov. 18th, 1933, had deep X-ray treatments at the Kingston General Hospital, left breast cycle. In autumn of 1934 noticed neuritis in left leg. Constant pain began in Feb., 1935. Pathological fracture July 3rd, 1935. Left leg is drawn up, shortened 3", undue motility, pain on pressure over great trochanter. Had deep therapy in Toronto. In July, 1935, was told nothing more could be done. Returned home in hopeless condition. Severe pain not controlled by narcotics. Was in moribund condition when admitted July 26th, 1935. First treated with Ensol July 26th, 1935. Pain was at once lessened. By Aug. 12th there was no bone pain and general condition was good. Oct. 15th, feels well. Oct. 27th, very well. In Nov. continued to improve. Jan., Feb. and March, 1936, continued to improve. April at home. May on treatment again. Improved. Oct. 5th to 18th, 1936, treated, very well.

Summary of X-ray reports July 26th, 1935 – Marking on both sides of chest are in favor of beginning secondary malignancy of both lungs with lymphatic permeation. Well marked secondary malignancy in the upper part of the shaft of the left femur, both trochanters, the neck and head of the bones. A pathological fracture of the neck is present. Also secondary involvement of both hip bones and head and greater trochanter of the right femur. Pelvis has a marked lateral tilt to the left side of alignment of spine.

Aug. 19th, 1935 – The neck of the left femur, the trochanter, the upper part of the shaft of the femur, all take part in the formation of a bow, with the trochanter surmounting the top of the bowed portion of the femur. There is a suggestion of a crack across the upper end of the femur whereas the previous break noted in the neck appears to be healing. It is also noted that the cortex of the lesser trochanter has been partially torn off. In addition to this it is noted that on the right side, where formerly there was seen radiolucent shadows in the head of the femur and the great trochanter suggesting rather large areas of metastatic destruction of bone, there are now seen only a few small areas suggesting metastases. It does not seem possible that the metastatic destruction previously noted could have been repaired during so short an interval of time, and I am rather of the opinion that the films are misleading in this respect.

Sept. 10th, 1935 – There is no evidence of either advanced or regression of the lesion.

Sept. 25th, 1935 – The pathological fractures of the upper end of the left femur are again noted. Both of these fractures have united with callus formation. There is, I believe, little evidence of new bone formation throughout the neck and great trochanter. Throughout the rest of the bones there does not appear to be any evidence of either progression or regression of the areas of secondary malignancy previously observed.

Oct. 11th, 1935 – The fractures of the neck and upper end of the shaft of the left femur are again seen, and at this time appear to have united with good callus formation. Throughout the upper part of the femur new bone is beginning to form replacing the radiolucent areas of malignancy. Other bony parts show no evidence of definite progression or regression.

Nov. 12th, 1935 – The old fractures of the upper end of the left femur are again observed, they are well united, and the deposits of secondary malignancy in the bone have pretty well faded out, leaving well-formed bone as the result. The neck of the femur has, however, not cleared quite as well in this process as the other parts, and I believe that another treatment with X-ray over the neck of the femur would be useful. Observation of the other femur and of the pelvis shows neither regression nor progression of the secondary malignant changes in the bone, this being at the end of four months since the first film was made. The head of the right femur is flattening a little, apparently due to the fact that the patient is now putting some weight on the softened bone.

Dec 10th, 1935 – The old fractures of the upper part of the left femur are now well united with good callus formation, and new bone is seen filling in the areas destroyed by secondary malignancy. Observation of the right hip shows that the secondary malignancy in the femur and the adjacent portions of the pelvic bone has advanced unfavorably.

Jan. 13th, 1936-It is noted that there is a spread of the malignant condition of the bone around the sacrum and the lumbar spine is tilted a little. In addition to this the head of the left femur is now becoming quite radiolucent. There is secondary malignancy of the head of the right humerus, of the scapula and of the clavicle.

March 27th, 1936 – The secondary malignancy of the bones previously noted is again seen. There is evidence of a little improvement following radiation; the bones being better calcified than previously.

May 27th, 1936 – There is evidence of re-calcification of bone of the head of the humerus, of the scapula and of the outer end of the clavicle. In the pelvis, re-calcification of the bone of the secondary malignant areas is again seen and remains about the same as on March 27th.

Oct. 5th, 1936 – Some improvement noted in the secondary malignant condition of the bodies of the spine. Dorsal spine shows increased calcium content. There is evidence of unfavorable progression in both trochanters and in the shaft of the right femur-also in the lower end of each femur and upper end of the tibia. The shoulders are not changed in appearance. Chest film suggests beginning secondary malignancy of the lungs of the lymphatic permeative type. (Compare this with statement in first report, July 26th, 1935, one year and three months earlier.)

Record of Deep X-ray Therapy Mrs. R.B.S.

1933, Sept. 9-13 – Left breast cycle.

Nov. 16-18 – Left breast cycle.

1935, July 26-27 – Left hip area.

Nov. 14-21 – Both hip regions.

Dec. 11-13 – Right hip region.

1936, Jan. 14-20 – Cervical spine, right shoulder, left shoulder, lumbar spine, sacrum.

Feb. 7 to March 15 – Both hips.

March 30 to April 2 – Left and right shoulders.

July 21-25 – Cervical spine and right thigh.

Oct. 6-16 – Cervical spine, both thighs and knees.

Comment This case is fully reported for several reasons. It was an early case, No. 28. It had been abandoned by the radiologists, and was moribund at home and suffering intense pain in spite of narcotics. It was brought to hospital to receive Ensol treatment. It was decided to employ deep X-ray therapy as well. It has received both Ensol and deep X-ray for a year and four months. There was, under the combined treatment, immediate improvement with control of pain. General condition improved until the patient was walking again and partly resumed her usual life. The radiologist has openly stated that any improvement that took place in this patient was due to radiation alone and the films have been exhibited to illustrate very remarkable regeneration of bone in secondary malignancy under radiation. However, it is a case of combined treatment that was about to die. The outcome has been most unusual and remarkable. After all, it is not important to apportion the credit. It is merely suggested that as those who are investigating the value of Ensol insist that all other accepted forms of treatment be employed; the radiologists and surgeons should be willing to add Ensol to their resources to learn whether it may not be to the advantage of their patients. Surely the welfare of the patient is the ultimate objective.

Case 28 S.C., age 57. Carcinoma, oesophagus.
Clinical diagnosis. First symptoms July, 1932, slowly increasing dysphagia. Now has difficulty with solids. Had 14 deep X-ray treatments (Western Hosp., Toronto). Admitted July 30th, Ensol used from that date to June, 1936. Aug. 3rd, swallowing much better. Aug. 7th, eating improved, gain in weight 5 1/2 lbs. Aug. 15th, generally better, weight 122 1/2 lbs. Aug. 30th, better, weight 123 1/2 lbs. Sept. 7th, swallowing improved, feels well, further gain in weight. Oct. 14th, improved. Nov., home with Ensol to be used by Dr. R.R. Nov. 23rd, able to eat all foods, weight 123 lbs. Nov. 30th, feels fine. Dec. 18th, well, working hard, eats all foods. Jan. 10th, 1936, developed bronchitis. Jan. 12th, severe cough, bringing up pus. Jan. 14th, losing weight. Jan. 18th, X-ray shows chest clear. Jan. 23rd, cough worse, rales throughout chest. Jan. 28th, takes about five glasses of liquids per day but losing weight. Feb. 19th, taking more nourishment. Feb. 28th, downstairs, feels stronger, slight traces of pus expectorated, weight 105 lbs. March 22nd, gain 22 lbs., at work daily. March 26th, husky, cachexia increased. March 31st, treated at office, eating mashed potato, bread. April 18th, weight 109 lbs., eating bread, potato, chopped meat, working. May 13th, unable to swallow water. May 16th, not swallowing, coughed up dark blood and tissue. May 27th, not swallowing, glucose

per rectum. June 5th, some bleeding. June 9th, operation, gastrostomy, doing well for two days, developed pneumonia. Died from pneumonia. Post Mortem – No enlarged glands. Gland from stomach region showed no carcinoma.

Dr. R.'s comment "All hope of this patient was given up in January. No other form of treatment would have done so well."

Case 135 Mrs. M.deM., age 67. Epithelioma of Vulva.

June 20th, 1935, excised. Aug., 1935, recurrence in scar. Aug. 22nd, 1935, first treated with Ensol. Nov., complete disappearance of growth. April, 1936, no sign of recurrence. Dr. C. writes, Nov. 30th, 1935, "This was in my opinion a very hopeless case of recurrence of epithelioma of the vulva, and she has now no trace of its macroscopically." April 11th, 1936, "This patient remains free from any detectable sign of recurrence. She has also increased in weight about five pounds." Nov., 1936, no recurrence.

REGIONAL DISTRIBUTION OF
PRIMARY MALIGNANT TUMOR IN 774 CASES
Prepared by G.S.B., MD

Breast	195	24%
Stomach	79	10
Rectum	78	10
Uterus and Cervix	76	10
Colon	50	7
Ovary	41	6
Prostate	36	5
Skin	29	4
Oesophagus	25	3
Lung and Pleura	15	2
Bone	15	2
Glands in neck	15	2
Larynx	12	1.5
Tongue	12	1.5
Pancreas	11	1.4
Lip	9	1.2
Nasal Sinuses	8	1.2
Urogenital Sys. (Kidney, Bladder, Urethra, Testes, Penis, Vulva)	33	4
Miscellaneous (Liver, undiagnosed primary, Thyroid, Parotid, Brain, Eye)	35	4
Total	774	

In 716 cases of cancer there was a positive history of malignancy in 213 or 29.7%.

This is probably not the actual total percentage as in many cases the patients did not know whether or not members of their families had been victims of cancer.

These figures are prepared from cases of cancer admitted to the Kingston Clinic between Aug. 1, 1935 and Oct. 31, 1936.

SUMMARY OF RECENT CASES

G.S.B., MD

From May 1st to Oct. 30th, 1936, many cases applying for treatment were rejected by correspondence as they were obviously in the very late stages of the disease.

One hundred and fifty cases were admitted to the clinic and of these fifty-six were not treated. Three were found to be not malignant; in six treatment was postponed and two were sent home with Ensol to be used by the attending physician. The remaining forty-five were so hopeless and far advanced they were advised to return home.

Of the ninety-four cases treated eighty-three were also advanced, all had received all the benefit possible from surgery, X-ray and radium. They had been told that nothing more could be done for them. Of these eighty-three, twenty did not respond to treatment or appear to be changed or benefited by it during the period they were under observation. Sixty-three responded to a greater or less degree, varying from mitigation of severity of symptoms to definite progress towards recovery of good health.

These figures indicate that Ensol treatment is still being utilized almost entirely among those abandoned to die in the very near future. For research purposes it is an excellent field of work and it is a great satisfaction that so much has been done for them. Some observers have advanced the statement that remedy such as Ensol should "cure all" cases. We are not so optimistic. When tissue has been destroyed and function seriously impaired, there is no possibility of recovery.

Attention is again directed to Case 8 narrated fully in Bulletin No. 1.

The patient was a man of 80 years of age. Clinical diagnosis was made of carcinoma of the stomach. Operation was contraindicated by age and general condition. No radiation was given.

Ensol was first used on July 19th, 1935. By July 27th he had stopped vomiting, was eating three ordinary meals a day and had gained three pounds in weight. Under continued treatment with Ensol alone his condition steadily improved and the mass in the abdomen had disappeared entirely by September. He remained in good health till December when he took cold and died on December 29th, 1935. The cause of death was stated to be a failing heart with early broncho-pneumonia and oedema of the lungs.

83

In the summary of the case, the pathologist begins with *"Atrophic Carcinoma of the Stomach."* In the discussion he adds, *"the cells found in the greatly thickened floor did not show definite cancerous features."*

What is the significance of these statements?

Did Ensol produce the atrophy?

If not, what did?

From the contents of these bulletins the reader will easily follow the advance of the constant research which was taking place and learn first hand the results of treatment of cancer patients by their attending doctors in different parts of Canada, the USA, and Australia.*

The information contained in the detailed and carefully prepared case histories shows the interest, concern and support of those many doctors treating varied types of cancer.

During the years 1935 through 1938 the work of the Foundation on cancer research expanded and the production of Ensol was increased to meet the continuing interest and requests for the serum from a constantly growing list of practitioners and patients.

*Complete bulletins available, see appendix.

HENDRY-CONNELL RESEARCH FOUNDATION
Kingston, Ontario, Canada

H.C. CONNELL, BA, MD, CM, *President and Director*

G.S. BURTON, MD, CM, *Director, Kingston Clinic*

G.A. CONNOLLY, MD, *Director, Wilmington Clinic*

B.J. HOLSGROVE, *Director of Laboratory*

J.C. CONNELL, MA, MD, CM, LL D, *Editor*

Editorial from Bulletin No.3

It has often been stated that no kind of internal medication can have any influence in limiting cancer growth, much less in causing its disappearance. Not long ago a surgeon, distinguished in cancer work, stated publicly that no cure for cancer would ever come out of a bottle. Yet this may prove to be another of the many impossibilities which have become realities in our own generation. To deny the existence of a chemical remedy for cancer is merely an attitude of skepticism which would deny it a fair trial when discovered. A large section of the medical profession, including many surgeons and radiologists, have declared such disbelief. On the other hand, there are research workers, clinicians, surgeons and radiologists who are seeking a chemical remedy for cancer, who continue to explore the frontiers of knowledge, with open minds and with confidence that sooner or later difficulties will be overcome and a useful chemical method of treatment developed. Inadequacy of present methods of treatment by surgery and radiation and the deficiencies in laboratory diagnosis of cancer are universally recognized. These conditions should stimulate the search for other means of diagnosis and treatment and render the profession responsive to evidence of advances. It is scarcely necessary to allude to the importance of an effective biochemical treatment that can be placed in the hands of the general practitioner as well as those of the surgeon and radiologist. Early treatment at home by the attending physician in addition to the use of surgery and radiation, when these are indicated and available, ought to reduce the mortality from malignant disease. It is noted, however, that many expect a chemical remedy to be a "cure" if its use is to be countenanced, regardless of the nature, duration and extent of the malignant disease. So-called trials of a remedy have been made when cases were within a few days or weeks of termination and then reports returned that no benefit was observed from the use of such treatment – a statement equally true for any remedy for any disease when administered too late to be effective.

Surgery versus Radiology

History repeats itself and will continue to do so, since human nature remains the same throughout the ages. Scarce twenty years have passed since the opposition of surgeons to the use of radiation in the treatment of malignant diseases was broken down. The new generation of radiologists is reminded that friendly relations with surgeons were a slow growth. The quotation below was written more than ten years after it became known that radiation was of use to control malignant disease.

> **From the Memoirs of Sir Almeric Fitzroy, Clerk of the Privy Council.**
> I have been obtaining information for the Prime Minister on the subject of a Royal Commission on cancer. Lords Lister and Rayleigh were the obvious people to appeal to, though in the present state of medical opinion nothing but a dubious judgment could be expected. Lord Lister wrote very courteously but expressed nothing more than the opinion of the medical authorities, which I knew would be unfavorable to investigations by any independent body. Lord Rayleigh disclaimed any qualification to speak on his own responsibility, but undertook to ascertain whether the Council of the Royal Society would advise on the point. The medical profession will hear of nothing but the surgical treatment of cancer, partly because of its traditional repugnance to the introduction of new methods and possibly owing to the enormous profits that accrue from operations for cancer.
>
> Jenner, Simpson, and to a lesser extent, Pasteur and Lister, have all in turn had to encounter the opposition of the Mandarins of the profession.

The radiologists triumphed and now there is the same form of compact between the present occupants of the citadel to resist encroachment upon their profitable field of operations and radiations. But the final result will be the same because something more must be added to their resources to overcome the ravages of cancer.

It was fortunate for humanity that radiologists persisted in the study of the action of X-rays and radium and prevailed over illogical prejudice and so-called vested interests among the surgeons. Had the opposition views been accepted and radiation discarded and discontinued the loss inflicted upon the world would be very great indeed. It is well that there are always within the profession some minds not atheromatous with the toxins of the text books. The orthodox of today are the heretics of yesterday. If history teaches one thing more than another, it is to beware of dogmatism and intolerance.

Clinical Research

There are some who hold that no clinical use should be made of any remedy until its action has been fully demonstrated in the laboratory. Experimentation upon patients has been condemned recently when the use of Ensol was being reviewed. Such an attitude might be justified if the practice of medicine were an exact science and not essentially experimental. Research in its most lowly form is employed constantly by all practitioners. How often does the doctor hand a bottle of medicine or a prescription to a patient and remark, "Try this and if you are not better come back and I will give you something else." Compare that with the exact administration of a new remedy under conditions which provide accurate observation and estimation of its effects. When preparations have been proved harmless to normal tissues and functions they should be used clinically under proper supervision. Close association between laboratory and clinic makes for progress. In this case, if the bacterial filtrate known as Ensol had not been used clinically in the human patient it could never have been discovered that pain alleviation is an outstanding effect of its use. Medical research confined to the laboratory has been greatly overdone while the clinical aspects of problems have been neglected. How relatively few are the workers in the field of clinical research.

Independent Clinical Reports

About one thousand patients have been treated with Ensol under immediate supervision at Kingston. Over three hundred and fifty independent physicians have administered Ensol to their own patients at home. So that the total number of patients treated approximates two thousand. This is increasing every day. These physicians are scattered all over this continent and in Australia, Hawaii and Cuba. Few of them are known personally to any of the staff of the Foundation. The Ensol was sent out, without charge, on the sole condition that short case histories and progress notes would be sent in for the records of the Foundation. Their clinical observations following the use of Ensol correspond to those at our own clinic. The results of treatment are so constant and consistent that they cannot be regarded as accidental or fortuitous. A few of these independent physicians were invited to report a case for use in this Bulletin and, with one or two exceptions, all responded. They appear elsewhere in this issue. There can be no doubt but that the improvement in these cases was due to the treatment and not because of other factors. If only a small number had been treated and a few had responded it would be unwise to report only these. So many have been treated it is no longer possible to report them all though the records of all are available. Many cases on the verge of death were treated in the hope that some mitigation of suffering or slight prolongation of life might ensue. In many such cases that hope was realized since they experienced marked alleviation of the pain from which they had been suffering. Of course these cases had received all possible benefit from surgery and radiation and, having been abandoned, were forced to narcotics for relief of pain. Such relief is partial, temporary, calls for constantly increasing dosage – in effect, has all the disadvantages associated with the use of narcotics. Any remedy which will replace narcotics in such cases and render their use unnecessary is valuable indeed. That Ensol does this is undoubtedly the case.

Thanks are due to the physicians – radiologists and surgeons among them – far and near, who have expressed confidence in and given support to the work of the Foundation. That there have been so many is a matter of surprise and satisfaction. Any one who ventures into the clinical field of cancer research in these days is immediately under suspicion and accused of ulterior motives. But that risk is of little account. Real progress can only be made by close cooperation between laboratory and clinic.

All who have worked with this Foundation and all who have in any degree received benefit, are under deep obligation to the sponsor who has generously contributed to its support. Without his benefactions progress would be slow indeed. It is due to his liberality that Ensol has been so widely distributed, without charge, over so long a period. The Wilmington Clinic has always been free. Recently it became possible to make the Kingston Clinic free also. The total amount of Ensol sent out free up to February 28th, 1938, is 125,351 cc's.

CHAPTER 5

After a little over two years of an exceptional relationship with Dr. Ellis Macdonald and the Franklin Biochemical Research Foundation in Philadelphia, tragedy struck the whole cancer research project which was to have the most devastating results for both the Kingston and Philadelphia laboratories.

A shipment from the Philadelphia laboratory received by Dr. T.A. Neal in Orlando, Florida was somehow contaminated, and resulted in the tragic deaths of ten of his patients during a period of one week, during the last days of March and the first days of April, 1938.In the past these same patients had been successfully and safely treated with both Ensol and Rex (the product from Philadelphia).

The news of this tragedy hit the papers all over the continent (Washington, New York, Philadelphia, Chicago, Toronto, Ottawa and of course in Kingston). Dr. Connell did all in his power to alleviate the frantic fears of all other patients. There was instant recall of all shipments and vials of serum in the hands of 149 doctors all over the continent. Investigations began in Orlando and also in Kingston and Philadelphia.

An article in the *Kingston Whig-Standard*, Wednesday, March 30, 1938, with large headlines reads as follows:

SIX DIE IN FLORIDA FOLLOWING ENSOL INJECTIONS

Ensol Deaths Not Fault of Local Laboratory

CHICAGO, MARCH 30-(AP)

Dr. Morris Fishbein, spokesman for the American Medical Association announced today six persons had died in Orlando, Florida in the last 24 hours from the effects of "Ensol" manufactured in Kingston, Ontario, Canada as a cancer treatment, and which apparently had become "contaminated". Two other persons were critically ill, said Dr. Fishbein, editor of the Association's Journal.

He said symptoms were similar to those of lockjaw. Dr. Fishbein said the drug known as Ensol was manufactured in Kingston, Ontario and was introduced in September 1935.

Dr. Fishbein said the cases would be investigated by the Federal Food and Drug Administration and the United States Public Health service. Investigators obtained samples of the drug used at Orlando. Dr. Fishbein said for bacteriological examination.

He added that he did not expect deaths would be widespread, since the product, because of its manufacture outside the country, would have only limited distribution here.

It is administered only by a physician, is not sold to the public across the counter and its sponsors claimed no uses for it other than cancer, Dr. Fishbein said.

DIED SINCE MIDNIGHT

ORLANDO, Fla., March 30-(CP)

Six women have died here and four other persons have been stricken with tetanus in the past 24 hours following injections of "Ensol" in treatment for cancer, President H.A. Day of the Orange County Medical Association disclosed today.

Dr. Day said the six deaths had occurred in Orlando hospitals since midnight. They and the four who are in serious condition were stricken with tetanus (lockjaw) yesterday.

Dr. Day said in every case death came much sooner than usual in tetanus cases.

Dr. Day said every effort was being made to locate all persons who had received the injection treatment for cancer. He declared the serum used in the cases which had proven fatal came from the office of a physician here. Most of the injections, he said, were administered Saturday.

The County Medical Association president requested the State Board of Health to send representatives here to aid outopsies. He also notified the American Medical Association of the deaths.

Coroner Eugene Duckworth said he would name a jury of "leading citizens to make a thorough investigation." He had not set a time for the inquest.

Dr. Day explained the serum had been used here for some time with no ill effects reported.

INVESTIGATION ORDERED

WASHINGTON, MARCH 30-(AP)

The Federal Food and Drug Administration ordered an investigation today into the deaths of six persons at Orlando, Florida, which officials said had been attributed to a cancer serum manufactured in Kingston, Ontario. Doctors said the serum had become contaminated.

The Canadian legation here promised to co-operate in every way to obtain a list of sources to which the drug had been sent in the United States.

DR. CONNELL

Dr. Hendry Connell made a statement this afternoon in connection with the reported deaths at Orlando, Fla., of six persons who have died in the past twenty-four hours, and all of whom had been given recent injections of "Ensol", a substance used in the treatment of cancer and prepared at the Hendry-Connell Research Laboratory in this city. The symptoms of those people who have died at Orlando are said to be similar to the symptoms of tetanus.

Dr. Connell declared he had been in telephone communication with Dr. Neal of Orlando, the physician who has been using Ensol and that Dr. Neal had told him the infection had been traced to one tube of Ensol.

Everything that leaves this laboratory has been checked and rechecked and there is absolutely no chance that there could be anything harmful in the Ensol that leaves here, said Dr. Connell. "This drug has been in use for three years and during that time 125,000 cubic centimeters have been used without any harmful results up until these cases in Florida. It is some local infection there and has no more than a chance connection with Ensol. It might have happened to anyone anywhere taking anything. Somehow these patients have become infected. Perhaps one tube of the Ensol has been contaminated but if this has happened it has been since the Ensol left the laboratory. "I can state definitely that there is absolutely nothing in Ensol manufactured here that possibly could have caused the deaths in Florida."

90

Also on Friday, April 1, 1938, *The Kingston Whig-Standard* reads as follows:

Discoverer of Ensol Offers His Aid

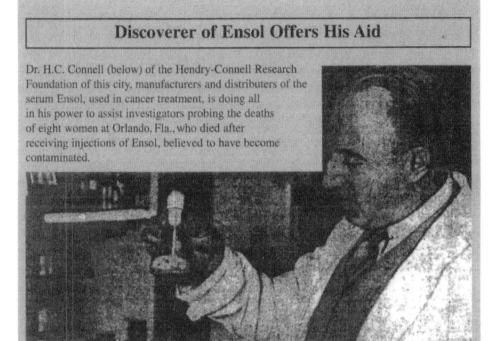

Dr. H.C. Connell (below) of the Hendry-Connell Research Foundation of this city, manufacturers and distributers of the serum Ensol, used in cancer treatment, is doing all in his power to assist investigators probing the deaths of eight women at Orlando, Fla., who died after receiving injections of Ensol, believed to have become contaminated.

And on the same page *The Kingston Whig-Standard* continues:

Orlando Death List Is Now Up to Nine

Man and Woman Die Today – Had been Injected With Cancer Serum – Inquiry Continues.

ORLANDO, Fla., April 1 (AP) A man and a woman died in hospital early today, bringing to nine the number of persons who have succumbed after being injected with a Canadian-made cancer treatment serum.

Mrs. Lydia Morrison, 49, and C.S. Pore, 65, both of Orlando, died within two hours of each other.

Six women died Wednesday and another yesterday and two other patients - a man and a woman - stricken at the same time were gravely ill today.

Ban on Ensol

OTTAWA, April 1 (CP) Distribution of Ensol has been prohibited until the National Health Department completes its investigations and tests now being conducted, Health Minister Power told the Canadian House of Commons this afternoon.

The *Philadelphia Inquirer / Public Ledger* reported on Sunday Morning, April 3,1938, the following:

TEST BEAR POISON IN CANCER SERUM: TENTH VICTIM DIES

ORLANDO, Fla., April 2 (AP) Dr. Horace Asa Day, president of the Orange County Medical Society, announced today laboratory experiments had proved tetanus toxin was present in two vials selected at random from a shipment of cancer serum received here by Dr. T.A. Neal, ten of whose patients have died in the past four days.

Dr. Day said he, Dr. J.N. Patterson, director of the State Board of Health laboratory in Jacksonville and Dr. W.G. Workman of the United States Public Health Service gave serum injections to guinea pigs in reaching their conclusion.

Some of the guinea pigs were given the serum and anti-tetanus toxin simultaneously last night and some were given only the serum. Some which received only the serum injections were dead this morning, said Dr. Day, and others showed symptoms of tetanus (lockjaw). Those which also were given the anti-toxin were still alive, he said.

The result of the tests, said Dr. Day caused physicians to believe the entire lot of serum received by Dr. Neal had been contaminated by tetanus toxin. Previously it had been Dr. Neal's theory that only one bottle was contaminated.

All of the ten persons who have died and the four now ill showed symptoms of tetanus.

The death early today of E.F. Bolte, 70, retired president of the International Harvester Comany, increase the fatalities to ten.

Coroner Eugene Duckworth said Dr. Day reported to him the serum used in injections here was manufactured in Philadelphia by the Biochemical Research Foundation and was called Rex.

"I will ask officials of the Biochemical Research Foundation of Philadelphia, manufacturers of Rex under the Canadian Ensol formula, to come to Orlando to testify at the inquest", Duckworth said.

DENIES CONTAMINATION

Investigation of bacterial filtrate shipped from the Biochemical Research Foundation of the Franklin Institute, 36th and Walnut Sts. has revealed that it contains no contamination. Dr. Ellice McDonald, director of the Foundation, reported yesterday.

Tests of the shipments were ordered Friday following a report from Orlando, Fla., that some of the serum used at a cancer clinic there with fatal results came from the Philadelphia laboratory.

"Investigation in the laboratories here," Dr. McDonald said, "shows that our bacterial filtrate has no contamination. As a precaution in the interests of the public the lot under investigation has been recalled."

STATE TO SEIZE SERUM

HARRISBURG, April 2 (A.P.) - State Secretary of Health Edith MacBride-Dexter today ordered inspectors to every drug store in the State in search of cancer serum similar to that which caused 10 deaths at Orlando, Fla.

Dr. Dexter instructed the agents to concentrate in the Philadephia area, where a bacterial filtrate under investigation originated. "Any such serum will be confiscated," she said.

The *Philadelphia Record* also reports on Sunday, April 3, 1938:

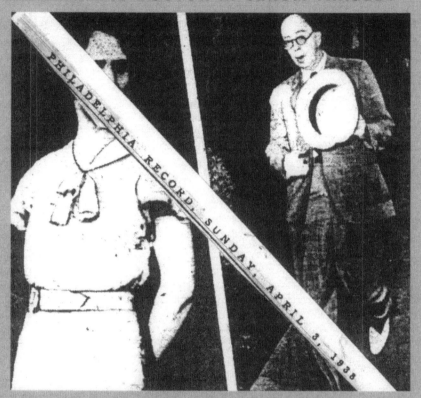

VICTIM AND DOCTOR IN SERUM TRAGEDY

Lockjaw Germs Revealed
In Test of Cancer Serum

**Tenth Patient Dies in Florida; Philadelphia
Laboratory Recalls Culture From Other Cities;
Insists Compound Was Pure.**

Tests of cancer serum shipped from Philadelphia to Orlando, Fla., revealed yesterday that it contained deadly tetanus germs.

That announcement was made by Dr. H.A. Day, president of the Orange County Medical Association, at Orlando, as a 10th cancer patient died there after serum injections.

From *The Morning Sentinel,* Orlando, Florida, Thursday, March 31, 1938.

*Cancer Serum Fatal For Six
Women,
With Doctors Fighting to
Save Others*

Ensol's Value Revealed
To Dr. Sinclair's Family

Ensol, serum for cancer, prolonged the life of the father of two Orlandoans, one a resident, the other a Winter visitor, it developed yesterday.

A contaminated serum which killed many Orlandoans this week and shocked two great sister nations of Canada and the United States, was brought home most forcibly to Dr. William Ewing Sinclair, M.D., and his brother Eldon Sinclair, of Toronto, the latter spending the Winter here.

Dr. Kenneth Sinclair of Toronto, a few hours from Kingston where the serum is manufactured, investigated the "cure" in 1934 and administered it to his father who died about a year after the treatment started.

"According to Dr. Kenneth Sinclair's brother, Dr. Sinclair of Orlando, their father was stricken with cancer of the throat in 1931 and suffered for three years.

Ensol was then being tested. It was commanding the attention of the Canadian medical world and profession.

"My brother, Dr. Kenneth Sinclair and my other brother, Eldon Sinclair, now spending the Winter in Orlando, went to Kingston, saw the serum in its processes of production, returned with some for my father," Dr. Sinclair related yesterday.

"For about a year father was given the serum. He was relieved and benefited but the throat infection had gotten too much of a start on us. He died when he was 72 years old but the Ensol remedy did not do it.

"It is my belief that the particular batch or bottle or shipment sent here was bad, that is, contaminated.

"It is possible that this batch of serum which came here and caused these deaths was due to cancer tissue serum with tetanus (lockjaw) serum in it, that is, from human cancer tissue infected with this bacilli.

"My two brothers personally investigated Ensol when it first came out. They went to see how it was administered and its effect. They were of the opinion that it was a good serum and would cure the disease if taken early. When I went to Canada I also gave it considerable study and watched the effect on my father. He seemed to be greatly relieved and helped but having had throat cancer for two years the new formula could not cure him.

INTO MUSCLES

"The Ensol is injected into the muscles, and from the muscular system it gets into the blood stream, seeks the infected spot. Usually one to two c.c. is given every day in the arm, preferably. This is repeated for some time or several days and then the treatment is stopped. The patient is closely watched. If there is a flare-up the treatment is again given.

"When I was in Canada several years ago the serum was comparatively hard to get because so many were pleading for it.

"I have heard some changes were made in the formula in recent months but am unable to say positively.

"The basis of the serum is an extract from cancer tissue.

FORMULA APPROVED

"For years this Dr. Connell who has been connected with the medical college at Queen's University at Kingston has been experimenting in cancer research. His formula was more or less approved by the Canadian medical association and profession but I am not sure on this point. I do not think the remedy has ever been approved by the American Medical Association.

"It is my understanding that in recent months the process has had something added to it, a form of antiseptic.

"Both my brothers have told me of the curative effect it has had. They recounted stories of the serum being tried in charity cases and on inmates at jails and prisons."

Dr. Sinclair said that old serum, that is, the serum injected into his father's arm was made from a bacillus proteus process.

In effect, the bacillus proteus was used on the cancer tissue and as a result liquid came from the tissue; the bacillus ate up the cancer tissue, left the serum behind. Great hunks of meat infected with cancer were hung up, the bacillus proteus placed on it for 24 hours, a clear liquid remaining which was the serum.

*Super-Horrible Agonies
Gripped Those Who Died*

"Patients who have died from Ensol have horrible deaths," eye-witnesses yesterday told the Sentinel.

"The respiratory organs cease to function and they die instantly.

"There is no way to describe the death except to say it is super-horrible.

"Their bodies get more or less rigid, their heads straighten and turn backwards.

"Then their jaws set.

"Their breathing becomes shorter.

"There is an upheaval in their chests.

"There is no death rattle.

"The respiratory system collapses.

"They are dead."

So run the stories from stunned nurses who have groped for restoratives.

Literally, they struggle to find words to describe their reactions to a most horrible death, used as they are to seeing humans slip into immortality.

In plain words the victims of this cruel, contaminated single batch of Ensol died of lockjaw.

In plainer words they suffered lockjaw, first, and suffocation, second.

The horrors of fatally wounded men on battlefields, or victims of wrecks, are concentrated in an Ensol death.

When nurses trained to death in all its multifold aspects shrink and shudder in describing an Ensol demise it surpasses description, reaches the perfection of human tragedy, crowns death in its most glorified terror.

Dr. Connell Satisfied One Bottle Was Contaminated

KINGSTON, Ont. – Dr. Hendry Connell, Kingston physician who discovered the Ensol treatment for cancer, said yesterday he was "ready and willing" to go to Orlando if necessary, to assist in investigating the deaths of six persons who died after taking it.

Dr. Connell has described his fluid as a protein product.

In a bulletin issued in January, 1937, he said it was not a cure and that its "present limitations are fully recognized, acknowledged and accepted."

"I have been in touch with an Orlando doctor and I am convinced one bottle of Ensol became contaminated after it left Kingston," Dr. Connell said. "Other bottles in the same shipment have been used at Orlando without harmful results."

Dr. Connell said he made a quick investigation in his laboratory and then telephoned Orlando.

"There can be no question that only one bottle was involved in the Florida cases," he said. "I am sure the Ensol contained in that bottle was not contaminated before it left here. It might have become contaminated in several ways."

Dr. Connell said 125,000 bottles of Ensol had been shipped to various parts of the United States and Canada since he announced discovery of the treatment in July, 1935. He said all had been sent free to clinics "interested in using it for treatment of cancer."

Dr. Connell, an eye, ear, nose and throat specialist, discovered Ensol in Queen's University Laboratories and announced it first July 17, 1935.

He said then he realized his announcement might be regarded as premature but his laboratory findings were positive and conclusive and early clinical effects uniform and "remarkable."

In October, 1935, Dr. Connell's report of his discovery in the Canadian Medical Association Journal told of 29 persons, all given up to die of cancer, who were injected

intra-muscularly with his digestive fluid from May to August, 1935.

The report said two apparently recovered, four died, five were relieved of all pain, the pain of nine others was diminished, and the cancerous growths of a number of others appeared smaller.

He said there had been no harmful reactions among patiens at the Kingston Clinic to whom more than 25,000 injections had been given.

City Health Physician Asks For Calmness in Tragedy

City Health Physician Claude Anderson yesterday called upon the people of Orlando to veer from hysteria over the wave of deaths resulting from the cancer treatments. Following a session of the City Board of Health, which was attended by Dr. Neal, Dr. Anderson issued the following statement:

"We have just had a meeting of the Board of Health. People have the wrong idea about these deaths.

"There is no epidemic of lockjaw in Orlando.

"The whole gist of the matter is that Dr. Neal has been using a certain type of serum as a treatment for incurable cancer cases. According to the information available he has administered this to 12 people in Orlando. According to his statement six of these people have died and the other six have shown some symptoms of developing tetanus.

"The City Board of Health and the Orange County Medical Society have enlisted the aid of the American Medical Association in trying to trace any other serum which might be contaminated in other parts of the country."

Earlier in the day Dr. Horace

A. Day, president of the Orange County Medical Society, revealed that he had communicated with officials of the American Medical Association in Chicago by phone and that the association heads had contacted U.S. Public Health officials and members of the Pure Food and Drug Administration in furtherance of an exhaustive probe of the tragedies.

It was learned that the Pure Food and Drug Administration was making a strenuous effort to learn the names and addresses of persons who had been sent shipments of the drug in an attempt to retrieve all the Ensol now distributed about the country.

In a statement of Dr. Day to the press, he said: "We cannot say what is causing the death. However as all six persons dying went under identical conditions resembling tetanus, commonly called lockjaw, we are pretty thoroughly convinced the deaths are due from a faulty batch of the serum.

"A chemical analysis of the victims' blood and other organs which may be necessary, will be made. We are culturing the blood and spinal fluid for bacteria and hope to reach definite conclusions at an early date.

"The Orange County Medical Association is doing everything possible to get at the bottom of this dreadful thing, and will leave no stone unturned to reach a solution."

Treatment Leads To Horrible Death For Orlandoans

U.S. AIDS PROBE

Fatal Fluid Believed Contaminated With Tetanus Germs

Six persons, all of them women, were dead last night and doctors were battling in an apparently losing fight to save the lives of five others, all victims of a strange malady brought on by injections of Ensol, a cancer serum.

The dead were Mrs. Jack Sweetman, 42, 134 West Princeton; Mrs. L.J. Jackson, 44, 134 East Harvard; Mrs. W.R. Thompson, 70, 132 East Concord; Mrs. Elizabeth Fundeburke, 36 Palmer Street, all of Orlando, and Mrs. W.O. Braswell, 49, of Holopaw, and Mrs. H.V. Harnage, 24, of Route 1, Cocos.

Those expected to die at any moment were Mrs. Lydia Morrison, 908 Carter Street; Mrs. F.E. Moonert, Orange Avenue in Winter Park, and C.S. Pore of 803 East Amelia. Also fighting for his life was Edward F. Bolte of 7 Rose Arden Drive.

Mrs. Ola Hall of 113 North Hyer was in the Orange General Hospital with an acutely sore arm following an injection of the serum that was administered on Tuesday.

All of the other victims of the serum were given their shots last Saturday.

DEATH EXPECTED

Mrs. Morrison, 49, refused a second shot Sunday because of a sore arm. She was rushed to the Orange General Hospital Tuesday at 4:30 A.M. and hospital officials claimed that she might die at any instant.

Mr. Bolte, 70, retired sales manager for the International Harvester Company, was given but one shot of the serum Saturday and was admitted to the hospital yesterday. His condition was pronounced fair, but grave, late last night.

Mrs. Moonert, 65, and Mr. Pore, also about 65, were both given the shots Saturday and Dr. C.W. Lynn, head of the Florida Sanitarium where the pair were suffering agonies as their bodies were racked with pain as a result of effects of the drug, declared their chances for life were slim.

A twelfth patient, thought to have been given an injection of the deadly serum, could not be identified last night. Hospitals claimed that the persons named were the only victims of the drug being treated in the two institutions.

SYMPTOMS IDENTICAL

Symptoms noticed in each of the dead and dying were claimed by physicians working over the patients to be identical and pointed to tetanus (lockjaw) as a probable cause of death.

The serum, which had been administered in treating cancer for nearly three years apparently brought about a sudden and severe case of some disease closely akin to tetanus and resulted in the violent deaths of the six persons and untold agonies for those still suffering, doctors declared in describing the malady.

A coroner's jury, empaneled to study the wave of deaths in an effort to determine the exact cause last night had run into a definite snag when the six men learned that all six of the first drug victims had been embalmed before an autopsy could be performed.

Enraged when informed that the bodies had been hastily prepared for burial, Coroner Eugene G. Duckworth lashed out at Carey Hand, undertaker who handled four of the victims, and threatened him with arrest if he proceeded to embalm any subsequent bodies if the cause of death was obviously the serum.

96

A coroner's jury, composed of N.P. Yowell, foreman, H.N. Roth, Dr. Carl Hoffman, Dr. John Hatfield, Maynard Evans and Louis Dolive, was told by Duckworth that his secretary, Mrs. Alice Engdahl, had telephoned Mr. Hand and asked that embalming operations be held up pending an autopsy on at least one of the bodies.

"Mr. Hand replied that he was running his business and if any more bodies were brought to his funeral home that they, too, would be embalmed," the Coroner told the jury as it assembled yesterday afternoon preparatory to viewing the bodies.

"I tried to call Mr. Hand myself and had the phone hung up in my face," added Judge Duckworth.

"I have instructed both hospitals to hold any other bodies of victims of the drug until an autopsy can be performed.

"I don't intend to have any trouble in this investigation and I will put somebody in jail and I don't care who he is if my orders are not carried out," he added.

It was learned later that a Florida law passed in 1935 made it a crime for any undertaker to embalm any body where he had reason to believe that a crime might have been committed in connection with the death or where he had been warned by a coroner or physician to hold the body for a post mortem examination.

DENIES ASSERTION

Confronted with the assertion of Judge Duckworth, Mr. Hand denied that he had acted in violation of instructions, but had prepared the bodies for burial prior to any request to await an autopsy.

Both Mr. Hand and Dana Eiselstein of Eiselstein-Wigginton Funeral Home promised that no further victims of the drug would be embalmed until the coroner's jury had been notified and asked for instructions.

Additional difficulties were heaped on the jury when it was learned that three of the bodies of victims had been shipped out of town. Mr. Hand said that he had already sent the remains of Mrs. Harnage and Mrs. Braswell out of town for funeral services. Mr. Eiselstein advised the jury that he had sent the body of Mrs. Thompson to Jacksonville for burial and that the family of Mrs. Jackson had removed the body to the home for the night.

The jury adjourned after viewing the bodies of Mrs. Sweetman and Mrs. Fundeburke and will reconvene at 9 o'clock this morning to view Mrs. Jackson when her remains are returned to the Eiselstein-Wiginton Funeral Home for services.

PROBE PUSHED

Meanwhile, it was learned that members of the Orange County Medical Society and officials of the State Board of Health were pushing an examination to learn how the serum administered by Dr. T.A. Neal happened to be contaminated.

Dr. Neal, prominent Orlando physician and agent for Ensol, product manufactured by the Hendry-Connell Laboratories of Kingston, Ontario, Canada, and Philadelphia, Pa., claimed yesterday that he felt sure the bottle of serum used to treat twelve persons here on Saturday had been tainted.

"I have given fully 10,000 shots of the serum in the State during the past several years and have had wonderful results from the treatments administered," claimed Dr. Neal.

He said that he could not understand how the drug could possibly have become contaminated with fatal bacterial that caused the horrible deaths of the victims.

AIDED MANY

Dr. Neal, weary from three days and nights of sleepless vigil as he and a battery of other doctors and nurses battled to save the stricken victims of the injections, claimed that his cancer treatments with the serum had brought many advanced stages of the disease under control and had apparently aided in effecting cures in some of his patients.

It was learned that Dr. J.N. Patterson, director of the laboratory of the State Board of Health at Jacksonville, was in Orlando yesterday afternoon conferring with local medical authorities preparatory to conducting an analysis of the remainder of the drug in possession of Dr. Neal.

Judge Duckworth claimed that Dr. Neal had told him he had a quantity of the serum that he kept in a refrigerator and that he would turn the drug over to Dr. Patterson for testing purposes.

Dr. Patterson was working in cooperation with Dr. Horace A. Day, president of the Orange County Medical Society, and Dr. W.H. Spiers, president of the Florida Medical Association.

M.D. Rentz, joined by Lowrie M. Beacham, both investigators for the Pure Food and Drug Administration, cooperated with Dr. Patterson, Dr. Day, and other officials of the medical profession to conduct experiments with another bottle of serum received by Dr. Neal in the same package as that which he administered to the patients.

EXPLAINS PROCEDURE

Dr. Day explained procedure of the tests to the Orlando Morning Sentinel:

"Following a conference with Dr. Patterson, I find that samples of a vial of the serum with the same serial number and that came in the same package with that which was administered to the patients have been cultured for any possible type of bacteria.

"The remainder of this vial was hermetically sealed and given to agents of the Pure Food and Drug Administration to take to Washington for toxicological examination to determine whether there are any poisons in the serum.

"Time for reading of the bacteriological cultures of the patients' blood and the spinal fluid has not yet been sufficient for accurate diagnosis and the readings will probably be made some time Thursday or Friday," added Dr. Day.

TO INOCULATE ANIMALS

Dr. Patterson revealed last night that he would take a portion of the remaining serum back to Jacksonville with him for further experiments with injections into animals to determine the effect of the drug on the beasts.

Judge Duckworth indicated that the physicians would be called to testify in the inquest, date of which will not be set until the group meets this morning.

Ensol, the drug administered by Dr. Neal, was declared still in what virtually amounted to an experimental stage. The United Press quoted Dr. Morris

Fishbein, Chicago, editor of the American Medical Association Journal, as saying that the deaths in Orlando "followed advice of the official magazine of the American Medical Society against the use of it.

"The drug used at Orlando was a preparation developed at Kingston, Canada, against which we made specific warning at its first introduction," Fishbein said.

The journal editor also declared that a local investigation was being conducted in Orlando thru one of the society's doctors. Dr. Day is the person conducting the inquiry here for the American Medical Society.

SAME PROCEDURE

Word from Washington officials came to the effect that they would follow the same procedure they invoked several months ago when a large number of persons died over the nation from the use of Elixir of Sulphanilamide.

Dr. D.B. Dunbar, assistant chief of the Pure Food and Drug Administration in Washington, declared that Rentz and Beach, inspectors for the administration, were ordered here from Jacksonville.

Dr. Dunbar also said that an agent had been dispatched to the Canadian source of the drug and another to the Philadelphia outlet of Ensol. "We will drop everything else if necessary to confiscate the remainder of the drug in Orlando and other points of the nation," he told the press.

He said the Canadian Legation in Washington had promised that his country would make every effort to aid

in locating all shipments of Ensol in the United States.

Dr. Neal, in discussing the strange, but fatal, malady yesterday, claimed that he had placed high faith in the cancer remedy and said that the drug was more than just a method of relieving pain of those suffering from the malignant disease.

"I investigated the men who invented the serum and found them to rank high in the Canadian medical circles," he said. "They in turn investigated me and finally made me Florida agent for Ensol about two and a half years ago and I have been using the serum with amazing results ever since.

"I am sure the firm is very careful about putting the serum up. They check and double check each shipment and in a telephone conversation with the firm heads I was told that injections had been administered from the same batch that I received a portion of here and that no ill effects had resulted from the injections.

"They told me over the phone that injections ranged up to many times the strength of the shots I gave and had been administered from the batch of serum recently and that all the patients were apparently doing fine.

"I can't imagine what happened to the bottle of serum I received, it is tragic and awful and the worst thing about it is that the publicity which is bound to result may discredit what has been proven to me to be a definite aid to cancer victims."

Dr. Neal claimed that his faith in the serum was so great that he would not hesitate an instant to inject the serum into his own body if he should become afflicted with cancer.

Two days later *The Kingston Whig-Standard*, April 2, 1938, printed the following in large headlines:

FATAL CANCER SERUM WAS NOT FROM KINGSTON

Clear Bill Given
Dr. Connell
By Health Officials

Serum Used in Orlando, Where Ten Persons Died, Was Made in Philadelphia from Dr. Connell's Formula— Washington Official Expresses Relief at Clearing Up of Local Angle to Matter.

Florida Doctor Makes Explanation

ORLANDO, Fla., April 2- (AP) – E.F. Bolte, 70, retired vice-president of the International Harvester Company, died early today, increasing to 10 the number of deaths among a group of persons here given injections of a serum for treatment of cancer.

Bolte, who came from North Dakota, died while investigators of various agencies worked intensively to determine what caused the deaths. Eight of the previous victims were women.

Dr. W.G. Workman of the United States Public Health Service indicated the results of autopsies and analysis of the serum would be known shortly.

Meanwhile, four women were in a hospital with the same symptoms as those who died. Their condition was not critical, although anti-tetanus treatment was having little effect. Physicians said the symptoms were similar to those of tetanus (lockjaw)

except in the reaction to treatment.

Made in Philadelphia

Dr. T.A. Neal said 13 of those affected had been given injections at his clinic from a single bottle of the serum. He first said the serum was made at Kingston, Ont. Yesterday he declared he discovered he had used a serum made in Philadelphia.

Dr. Neal said he had used both serums in his treatment of cancer patients. The serums are identical, the Philadelphia preparation being made from a formula of Dr. H.C. Connell of Kingston.

Not Called Ensol

The serum made in Philadelphia, however, is not called Ensol, name of the product prepared in Canada.

Dr. Neal said that as soon as he suspected that it was the Philadelphia serum which was contaminated he inoculated mice with it. That was Thursday night and all the mice died yesterday, he declared.

In his treatment of patients, he had used both Canadian and United States manufactured serum. It was this circumstance which led to the confusion.

Dr. Connel's Statement

Dr. Hendry C. Connell said late yesterday he was "greatly relieved" to receive a

report from Dr. T.A. Neal of Orlando, Fla., that the serum which caused death to the Florida physician's patients had not come from Kingston.

Dr. Connell said he had been informed by Dr. Neal that the serum was not part of a Kingston shipment.

Dr. Connell said he had been told by Canadian authorities, who had been investigating the situation with United States officials, to continue shipments of Ensol but that he had held them up pending clean-up of the investigation.

Of the official inspection of his laboratory, Dr. Connell said: "We were given a clear bill by Dr. Harrison of the Health Department at Washington after he had been in touch with Washington following news that the serum used by Dr. Neal in Orlando was made in Philadelphia from our formula."

Dr. Harrison's Statement

American and Canadian health officials left Kingston Friday after conducting a two-day probe into the manufacture and distribution of Ensol at the Hendry-Connell Research Foundation laboratory. Dr. W. Harrison, of the National Health Institute of Washington told The Whig-Standard last night that he was satisfied with his investigation at the laboratory. He had given Dr. Connell a clean

99

bill of health. He had intended to leave for Ottawa last night to consult health officials there had not the information been relayed that the serum said to have caused deaths in Florida was manufactured in Philadelphia and not Kingston.

The three officials from the Dominion Department of Health returned to Ottawa early yesterday and Dr. Harrison said he had not seen them at all.

An American official from the food and drug administration of the Department of Agriculture, who had also come to Kingston, left yesterday at noon for United States.

"I am greatly relieved and very happy for Dr. Connell," said Dr. Harrison last night before he left. Although he had not been detailed by his Government to go to Philadelphia, he left for there last night. "We were informed by The Whig-Standard by telephone of the good news late in the afternoon before Dr. Connell received his telegram," explained Dr. Harrison. "The investigation just didn't seem to make sense from the first. Nothing like this had ever happened before. I made a thorough examination of the method of manufacture here and it only took a few hours. I am quite satisfied with everything here."

DepartmentRelieved

OTTAWA, April 2 (CP) Health officials were relieved last night when it was learned the cancer treatment serum from which nine persons were believed to have died in Orlando, Fla., was not Ensol from the Kingston, Ont., laboratory of Dr. Hendry Connell.

Three department officials who were sent to Kingston several days ago to investigate the manufacture and distribution of Ensol, returned to Ottawa yesterday.

Dr. W. Harrison, of the National Health Institute of Washington, a division of the United States Public Health Service, who was sent to Kingston at the same time as the Dominion Government experts, left yesterday for Philadelphia. It was believed the serum used in Orlando was manufactured in Philadelphia from the Connell formula.

Meanwhile the department here will complete its tests of Ensol, Health Minister Power said. Samples of Ensol were brought back from Kingston.

Mr. Power said Dr. Connell had given the department experts every assistance while they were making their inquiries in his laboratory.

Steps Being Taken

In the course of a statement to the House of Commons yesterday, Mr. Power described the steps taken by the Hendry-Connell Foundation to prevent further use of Ensol by those to whom it had been distributed, pending investigation.

"In the meantime," Mr. Power said, "all further distribution of Ensol has ceased pending results of laboratory examinations and autopsies."

In an interview last night, Mr. Power said:

"Our department officials consulted with Dr. Connell in Kingston when the deaths were reported and almost immediately he prohibited further distribution of Ensol and got in touch with persons whom he knew were using it as a treatment."

In his statement to the House of Commons Mr. Power said his department, under existing legislation, "is unable to supervise or control free distribution, as it has no authority therefore: nor has it authority to interfere with the making up and preparing of prescriptions by laboratories, by physicians themselves, or by hospitals."

"An application was made by the Hendry-Connell Research Foundation to manufacture and sell Ensol in 1935," he added. "A licence was refused and the applicant was advised that a licence would not be granted until such time as a pronouncement had been made upon the efficacy of Ensol by a responsible medical authority."

And from other cities in the USA:

LABORATORY IS ABSOLVED

Connell Research Foundation Exonerated of Blame in Serum Deaths

WASHINGTON, April 6. Dr. W.T. Harrison, chief of the biological division of the National Institute of Health, in a report to Acting United States Surgeon-General W.F. Draper last night, said that the "cancer serum" deaths in Orlando, Fla., last week were caused by a medicine manufactured in Philadelphia.

The report did not name the Philadelphia manufacturer, but it absolved the Hendry-Connell Research Foundation of Kingston, Ont., of any responsibility in connection with the deaths of the nine cancer victims who had taken the fatal serum treatment for their illness.

Dr. Harrison reported that an investigation disclosed the Philadelphia firm's product became contaminated with tetanus, or "lock jaw," germs during development of a cul

ture for the serum.

It was learned that the Philadelphia medicine, which was distributed at no cost to doctors for experimental purposes, was not licensed by the National Institute of Health. Officials, however, declined to discuss the matter.

It also was learned that Harrison had absolved the Philadelphia firm of any intentional guilt in the preparation of the serum.

SHIPMENTS LOCATED

DETROIT, APRIL 1-(CP) Three consignments of the cancer serum which has caused nine deaths in Orlando Fla., within a few days, were located here yesterday by Federal food and drug inspectors. Found among stock of two merchants and a physician, the shipments were set aside and samples taken for submission to Government Laboratories at Washington. One of the vials had been opened and half of its contents used, Inspectors said. There is a possibility the Detroit consignments might be part of that sent to Florida. It was being checked.

Three officials of the

Dominion Department of Health in Ottawa were sent to the Kingston Lab, also Dr. W. Harrison of the National Health Institute of Washington, a division of the Washington Public Health Service, and a representative from the Food and Drug Administration of the Dept. of Agriculture in the U.S.

All three Dominion Government experts had become satisfied and returned to Ottawa. Health Minister C.R. Power at the time said Dr. Connell had given every assistance while they were making their inquiries, and in his statement in the House of Commons April 1st, described the steps taken by

the Hendry-Connell Research Foundation to prevent further use of Ensol by those to whom it had been distributed. In the meanwhile Mr. Power said, "all further distribution and use of Ensol has ceased."

Before leaving for Philadelphia, Dr. Harrison said, "The investigation just didn't seem to make any sense from the first. Nothing like this had ever happened before. I made a thorough examination of the methods of manufacture, and it only took a few hours to be quite satisfied with everything here." Dr. Harrison stated that he was "greatly relieved and very happy for Dr. Connell."

101

During all this confusion and consternation in the Kingston lab on March 30-31, from Orlando there came a communication from Dr. Neal saying that the vial he had used had "not come from Kingston, but from the lab in Philadelphia." Dr. Neal said he had been using serum from the two sources and that is what caused the initial confusion for him. In the meanwhile, Dr. Neal, from the same vial, injected guinea pigs in their lab. The animals died the next day. Dr. Neal was then convinced that the vial from Philadelphia had been contaminated in some way.

It was not until Saturday, April 2nd, that these newspapers published the fact that the fatal serum was named Rex and produced in Philadelphia by the Biochemical Research Foundation of the Franklin Institute. Dr. Ellis McDonald, director of that Foundation was quoted as saying that his laboratory had been preparing and shipping their product since 1936 when they first started making the formula of Dr. Hendry C. Connell named Rex in the United States. In the Philadelphia *Evening Bulletin* of Saturday, 2nd April, 1938, there is a photo of Doctors J.J. Scanlon and L.C. Herring in Orlando searching for the cause of the death of ten cancer patients who received injections. In the same story it is reported that Dr. H.A. Day, president of the Orange County Medical Association at Orlando revealed that tests of the cancer serum shipped from Philadelphia contained deadly tetanus germs. Further to this same story, the Biochemical Research Foundation of the Franklin Institute is reported to have shipped a batch of serum to Orlando, March 22, and had meanwhile sent hurried orders for the recall of all serum made and shipped at that time. Dr. Ellis McDonald, director of the Foundation said,"Investigation in the laboratory here shows that our bacterial filtrate (serum) had no contamination. As a precaution, in the interest of the public, the lot under investigation has been recalled, however."

The Orlando paper of course, followed up the deaths more often and in more detail because of the very local interest. In columns adjacent to the reports of the ten deaths, there were a number of interviews with patients of Dr. Neal's who had been receiving injections of either Ensol or Rex over various lengths of time. Each patient interviewed reported a considerable degree of success and improvement, both in reduction or disappearance of pain, gain in weight and generally improved well being. Names and ages were given as well as specific problems. All

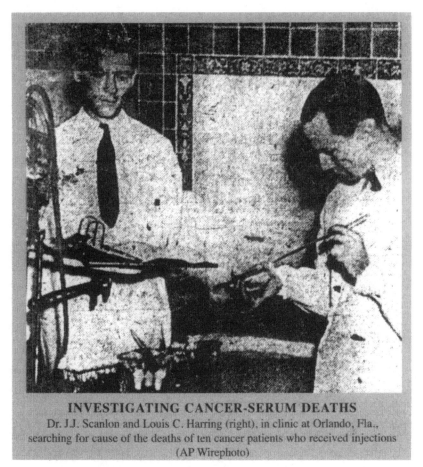

INVESTIGATING CANCER-SERUM DEATHS
Dr. J.J. Scanlon and Louis C. Harring (right), in clinic at Orlando, Fla.,
searching for cause of the deaths of ten cancer patients who received injections
(AP Wirephoto)

The Philadelphia Evening Bulletin, April 2, 1938.

expressed satisfaction and confidence in Dr. Neil's treatment and were prepared to continue with their treatment.

An inquest held in Orlando found the coroner's investigation frustrated because some bodies had been embalmed, buried or shipped to home towns where indicated. Research has not found any conclusion published. Reviews of the newspapers after the dates previously searched failed to find any further information or interest on this subject. It is not known when the production of Rex ceased, but the connection with Kingston appears to have stopped shortly after this episode, and those physicians treating cancer patients and submitting case histories, all referred to the product as Ensol instead of as Rex from that period on.

Form 8101, replacing Form 2A

CANADIAN NATIONAL
TELEGRAPHS

D. E. GALLOWAY, ASSISTANT VICE-PRESIDENT, TORONTO, ONT.

SERVICE DESIRED
Full-Rate Message
Day Letter
Night Message
Night Letter

Patrons should mark an X opposite the class of service desired; OTHERWISE THE MESSAGE WILL BE TRANSMITTED AS A FULL-RATE TELEGRAM

Exclusive Connection
with
WESTERN UNION
TELEGRAPH CO.
Cable Service
to all the World
Money Transferred
by Telegraph

RECEIVER'S NO.	TIME FILED	CHECK

Send the following message, subject to the terms on back hereof, which are hereby agreed to

27R CR 31   Ottawa, Ont 1147A April 8, 19 38

To Hendry Connell Research Foundation

Kingston Ont

Samples from Ansol batches ten one sixty eight ten one seventy
ten one seventy two ten one seventy five ten one twenty eight have
passed tests for sterility and tetanus toxin

R E Wodehouse Deputy Minister

1154 am.

104

CHAPTER 6

As a result of these newspaper stories, despite the very prompt work and clearance by the responsible authorities in Canada and the United States, the high reputation of the Hendry-Connell Research Foundation was severely damaged. The effect of the hasty and irresponsible reporting throughout the continent influenced many previous supporters who now feared and refused too close an association. Who knows what might have been the outcome if the work of the Foundation and treatment of patients had continued at the pace of the previous three years, if it had not been torpedoed in mid-passage?

The aftermath of this negative publicity soon became apparent.

Dr. Hendry Connell wrote to the Board of Trustees of Queen's University on August 31, 1938 on behalf of the Hendry-Connell Research Foundation as follows:

1. He requested an extension of the agreement dated 18th November, 1935 between the University and the Foundation be granted for either a three year period or on a year-to-year basis.
2. He also stated that the other conditions in the original agreement were satisfactory to the Foundation and expressed the appreciation of the Foundation for the assistance and support given so generously by the University and the hospital.*

In the course of discussion by the Board of Trustees to these requests, it was agreed that the university make no further monetary contributions directly or indirectly to the Hendry-Connell Research Foundation, but that the hospital be asked to renew for one year the use

*The Hendry-Connell Foundation, at their expense, had erected a temporary building costing about $10,000 on the grounds of the Kingston General Hospital. The site was granted by the hospital on the request of the university, and was to be vacated in three years. The time was now almost up. The university was supplying heat, light, gas and water at a cost of about $1,000 per year.

of the land on which the research laboratory stood. The hospital had stated that they desired to continue to act through the University and not directly with the Foundation. The board further decided that the university now go on record in stating that it had no responsibility for the work of the Foundation.

After this withdrawal of confidence and faith in the work of the Foundation by the University Board of Trustees, Dr. Connell was faced with another setback. The three-year agreement made in 1935 with the Franklin Institute was not renewed. In fact, the affiliation with the Biochemical Research Foundation of the Franklin Institute lasted only until January, 1938.

There is no indication of the Institute's acknowledgement of its responsibility for the deaths in Orlando.*

Effects

After the Florida affair there was a decrease in the support for the use of Ensol by skeptics and the university no longer wished to be closely connected with the Foundation.

A technician was reported to be taking off with the Ensol research: there is an affidavit signed in court reporting this action. This incident prompted the Foundation to draw up an agreement for all employees that they would not divulge any information about the procedures in the making of the enzyme solution. This agreement was put together by the Ontario Government and the board of the Foundation.

As the slowdown occurred, the most appreciated and valued secretary was given the opportunity to go to another job in Montreal with the CIL headquarters arranged by Dr. H.C. She became a valued and long time employee of that company.

Another episode was the making of a film by the Foundation showing a patient with a cancerous tumour of the outer ear, both before and after treatment with Ensol. The tumour became so small it was removed surgically at the Hotel Dieu hospital by a reputable surgeon. The tumour never returned. This movie was produced very professionally by Donald Alexander, the Foundation's chemist, in colour with good sound which at the time had to be processed in Toronto, as Kingston did not have facilities to coordinate pictures with sound. After being shown on many occasions, it was clandestinely removed from the

*All letters of enquiry are returned or not answered. Archives have no record – seems it's a closed book.

106

Foundation's office, and on thorough investigation, there has been no trace of it since.

During the financial distress it was a constant concern of Hendry's that the young professionals working for him should not be stalled in the advancement of their careers through a sense of loyalty. Eventually, when the time came for them to leave, it was always a wrench for these young people who had worked so hard and with such commitment.

All these problems seem the direct result of the erroneous newspaper reports that the contaminated vial was Ensol from the Kingston Laboratory rather than Rex from the Biological Research Laboratories in Philadelphia.

This immediately put a severe strain on the Foundation's finances, the continued research and the stated intention of providing Ensol free of charge to those patients being treated by their physicians.

Despite these upsets in a rapidly changing and war-threatened world, Hendry Connell had the confidence and faith of those many doctors in Kingston and beyond, who were having good results treating their cancer patients with Ensol, and consequently increased the demand for the product of the Foundation. As an example Dr. Walter Thomas Connell (no relation), Dr. Eugene Percy Jones and Dr. Robert Norton Irwin all travelled to Washington D.C. in late January 1941 to appear as witnesses in a civil action against the Commissioner of Patents. These three doctors as well as Hendry Connell upheld the findings in case histories over the last seven years that treatment of cancer patients with Ensol reduced or alleviated pain and suffering and prolonged life in a very high percentage of cases.

The outcome of this civil suit was that Ensol was patentable in the USA under that name.

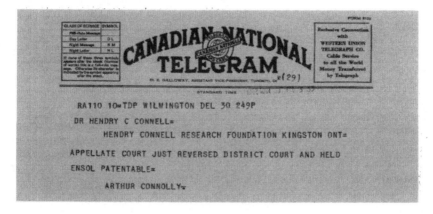

Patents

During the period from 1935 to 1939 more than twenty-two patents for Ensol were applied for and/or granted in countries around the world. This was a sensible precaution to protect the Foundation from any infringement of Ensol discovered and produced by the Hendry-Connell Research Foundation. The two most important of these patents were those granted by Canada and the United States. However, most of the European countries were included as well as Australia, South Africa, India, Japan, Ireland and Brazil. Russia was not included, as that country was not a member of the International Convention. These patents of course, would have had some considerable value if at any time in the future Ensol had been produced commercially. However, it was the aim of the Foundation and of the founders to provide Ensol free of charge to those suffering from cancer so long as such a goal could be maintained.

CHAPTER 7

CAPCO

When the money came from the Franklin Institute to assist in the research as had been arranged in 1935, it was transferred through a company called CAPCO to the Hendry-Connell Research Foundation.

It is of interest to know that Mr. Irenee DuPont was introduced to Dr. Ellis McDonald in 1927 and had become very much interested in his ideas of a chemotherapy approach to the cancer problem. Dr. McDonald, a Canadian, a graduate of McGill, was at that time professor of gynecology at the University of Pennsylvania Medical School. Mr. DuPont's grants of money for research were earmarked for Dr. McDonald's use, and when the Biochemical Research Foundation was established by Dr. McDonald as an adjunct of the Franklin Institute it was supported entirely by Mr. DuPont.

When Dr. McDonald became acquainted with Hendry Connell's work through the Franklin Institute, he likely told Mr. DuPont about Ensol because Mr. DuPont had his attorneys form the two CAPCO companies so that funds provided by him to assist Hendry's research could be transferred in exchange for shares to be made out to his favourite charities which would derive a source of income should the manufacture of Ensol become a profitable venture in the future. Certainly Mr. DuPont would be very familiar with patents and the various ways of dealing with each one, including the future prospects of any particular new invention or idea. It is interesting to speculate the present worth of such donated shares of actively successful companies now in the hands of charitable organizations. At that time the company slogan was, as now, *BETTER THINGS for BETTER LIVING ... THROUGH CHEMISTRY*, as shown at the bottom of the page of their letterhead in 1937.

CAPCO was a synonym for a corporation named Canadian-American Pharmaceutical Company. It was incorporated in Delaware on November 26, 1937. The certificate of incorporation was recorded with the Recorder of Deeds for New Castle County, Delaware, USA on December 1, 1937.

The Directors of the corporation were as follows:
Hendry C. Connell
Edwin B. Connolly
Arthur G. Connolly

This corporation was formed as a patent holding company only and the two Mr. Connolly's were attorneys-at-law in the Legal Department, Patents Division of the E.I. DuPont de Nemours & Company of Wilmington, Delaware.

The Officers of the corporation were:

Hendry C. Connell	*President*
James C. Connell	*Vice President*
Edwin B. Connolly	*Vice President*
Arthur C. Connolly	*Secretary Treasurer*

CAPCO (CANADA) was incorporated 5th July, 1938. The purpose and objective of this company was to "manufacture, buy, sell and deal in wholesale and retail, medicinal, chemical, biochemical, pharmaceutical and other useful preparations for scientific, medicinal and domestic use."

The directors of this company included some of the directors of CAPCO Inc.

At a special meeting on Wednesday morning November 29th, 1939 of the directors of the Hendry-Connell Research Foundation it was announced by the president that the funds were almost depleted. This was followed by a declaration that the Foundation would have to discontinue its present services to the public as well as all research from the last day of December, 1939.

The president announced that he had advised both Mr. DuPont and the Ontario Government of this serious condition by personal letter. Mr. DuPont had replied that he did not feel that it would be advisable to give further support to the research at present.

It was unanimously decided that H.C. Connell should go at once to Toronto to interview the Premier and the Minister of Health to inform them of this precarious financial position and ask them what the Government wished to have done. Dr. Irwin arranged an appointment for Thursday morning November 30, 1939. The eventual outcome of this meeting was a grant of $3,000 per month for, at that time, an undetermined period commencing January 1, 1940.

A further result of this meeting was that all connections with both the Canadian and American CAPCO organizations should be relinquished by all directors of the Hendry-Connell Research Foundation and if a licence should ever be issued to the Foundation the distribution commercially would best be left to a larger established house or houses under licence from the Foundation.

H.C. Connell met with Mr. Connolly in New York City on Thursday, January 11th, 1940 and all necessary business was completed and from that date the new plan was completed.

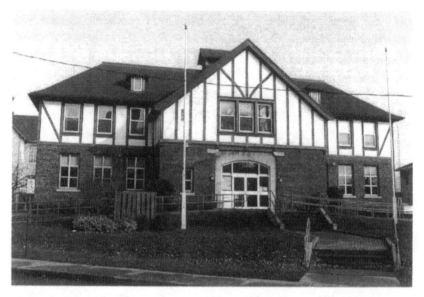

The present Barrie Street laboratory where the Cancer Commission of Ontario set up a research laboratory in 1938-40 to examine the Hendry-Connell Foundation's procedures in the production of Ensol

CHAPTER 8

MEMORANDUM RE ENSOL DEVELOPMENT
September 29th, 1939
H.C. CONNELL

No. 1

Early in 1938, the Ontario Government enacted legislation bringing all cancer remedies in the Province of Ontario under the control of the Ontario Cancer Commission.

Immediately following the appointment of the members of this Commission, the Hendry-Connell Research Foundation requested this body to undertake a survey of the work being carried on by them in the treatment of this disease.

On October 26th, 1938 the Commission gave the Foundation its first hearing. At this meeting the Commission accepted all the data presented and by mutual agreement appointed a sub-committee consisting of certain members of the Commission to visit the laboratory of the Foundation and view the work at first hand. The committee spent the day of November 18th, 1938 in Kingston.

The subsequent findings of the Cancer Commission which were passed on to the Government in December 1938, were as follows:

1. That the evidence to date shows that Ensol has been used fairly extensively for a period of three years.
2. That from the evidence to date Ensol was shown to be harmless when prepared, distributed and administered under rigid control.
3. That the Commission is not in a position to give final judgment on the clinical value of the preparation until work has been carried on under conditions to be laid down by the Commission.
4. That the Commission is of opinion that the Hendry-Connell Foundation has opened up a research problem with reference to Ensol and that the study of this problem should be continued.

113

The report of the sub-committee was adopted by the Cancer Commission.

The sub-committee included in their report the following clause:

Your Committee does not think it would be in the public interest to place Ensol on sale at the present time.

This report was issued on January 19th, 1939.

The Cancer Commission as a Commission did not include any recommendation against sale and the Chairman and a majority of the Commission were not in accord with the Commission saying or doing anything that would be construed as an expression by the Commission against the sale under licence from the Federal Department of Health. Any doubt in this matter can be readily cleared up by communication with the Chairman of the Commission, Mr. Justice Gillanders at Osgoode Hall.

On March 1st formal application for the granting of a licence to the Hendry-Connell Research Foundation was made to Ottawa by the Ontario Government through the Honourable Harold J. Kirby, Minister of Health, who wrote Honourable C.G. Power on March 1st, 1939 as follows:

Honourable C.G. Power, MC, KC,
Minister of Pensions and National Health,
OTTAWA, Ontario

Dear Mr. Power,
I hereby make formal application to your Department to have the Connell Research Foundation granted a licence to sell Ensol to physicians only. This application is made because we believe the product merits further clinical investigation and is now being used by numerous physicians who will be willing not only to pay for the cost of the Ensol but to report to the Connell Research Foundation the results obtained from its administration.

On March 6th, 1939 Honourable Mr. Kirby wrote the Honourable C.G. Power, the Minister of Health for the Dominion, the further following letter:

I wrote you under date of March 1st, regarding a licence being granted to the Connell Research Foundation to sell Ensol to physicians only.

I may say that in doing this we had in mind the unanimous opinion as expressed by the members of our Cancer Commission that Ensol has sufficient merit to warrant the Connell Foundation being encouraged financially in continuing its work. If it is to do this, it should be in a position to recover the cost of manufacture of the product from those physicians who are using it clinically, and your department has the authority to grant such permission.

Trusting that you will find yourself in a position to do so, I am,

Following this the Ontario Government decided to assist the Foundation in an extension of their laboratory investigation of Ensol by the appointment of suitable personnel to be paid for by and responsible to the Ontario Department of Health.

A formal agreement was entered into on behalf of the Province of Ontario by the Minister of Health for the Province of Ontario with the Foundation and duly executed.

Details of the agreement were carefully worked out and the Province on the one hand agreed to provide and pay certain trained persons and the Foundation on the other hand agreed in consideration of this assistance that during the continuance of the agreement the Foundation would provide Ensol and make Ensol available, free of charge, to physicians for the use in the treatment of their impoverished cancer patients who are residents of, and within the Province of Ontario.

Experts were at once appointed by the Government and approved by the Cancer Commission to carry on this work, such appointees being Dr. W.T. Connell, Dr. E.P. Johns and Dr. Beck. Dr. W.T. Connell has no connection with the Foundation nor any relationship with any member of it and the name is in this respect a mere coincidence. These men have completed and submitted a report definitely establishing the following facts:

1. Ensol is harmless and that it produces no undesirable immediate or remote effects.
2. In at least 65% of cases temporary systemic improvement is noted.
3. Local improvement is manifested by lessening of pain and tension and at times by definite shrinkage in the tumor mass.
4. Systemic improvement is seen in an increased feeling of well being, with improvement of appetite with consequent cessation of weight loss or actual gain in weight.

5. The local and systemic improvement is accompanied by a marked reduction in the necessity for sedatives and opiates.

A verbatim copy of such report dated 5th of September, 1939 is attached hereto for convenience.

These facts definitely established the present therapeutic value of Ensol in the treatment of disease.

All of which is respectfully submitted.

DATED this 29th day of September, A.D. 1939.

HENDRY-CONNELL RESEARCH FOUNDATION

H.C. Connell
President

MEMORANDUM RE ENSOL DEVELOPMENT
December 6th, 1939
H.C. CONNELL

No. 4

After due consideration by the Minister of Health and the Premier, it was decided that instead of a public announcement being made by the Minister of Health, it would be proper for the Minister to ask the Ontario Cancer commission to table in the House, a report on their work-to-date, on January 10th, 1940. As far as the Foundation is concerned this is quite satisfactory, provided of course, that the Commission's report will include the recent findings of Dr. W.T. Connell and Dr. Johns, bringing the work up-to-date at least as of December 15th, 1939.

Since the funds of the Foundation are almost depleted, and since there does not seem to be any disposition on the part of the Ottawa authority to grant a license for the sale of Ensol, the question of financial support for the Foundation has become acute.

This condition of affairs was brought to the attention of both the Ontario Government by personal consultation and to that of Mr. DuPont by a personal letter.

After consultation with Mr. Connolly, Mr. DuPont wrote me to the effect that he did not feel that it would be advisable to give further support to the research at present.

116

This meant that the Hendry-Connell Research Foundation would of necessity discontinue its present services to the public and also all research as from the last day of December 1939.

A special meeting of the Directors was called by me on Wednesday morning, November 29th, 1939.

After a very thorough discussion it was unanimously decided that I should go at once to Toronto to interview the Premier and the Minister of Health in order that I might inform them of the Foundation's precarious financial position and ask them what the Government wished to have done.

Dr. Irwin arranged an appointment for us with Mr. Kirby for Thursday morning, November 30th.

After discussion, it was felt that the Hendry-Connell Research Foundation should maintain its identity and that all its present activities should be kept up. In order that this might be possible the Government has promised a grant of $4,000 which it is expected will tide over the work till the end of January 1940. This was confirmed to me by letter from the Minister of Health, a true copy of which is here incorporated:

December 5th, 1939
Dr. H.C. Connell,
Hendry-Connell Research Foundation,
Kingston, Ontario.

Dear Dr. Connell:
Further to our discussion of Thursday last, might I say that in view of the Government's interest in not only the laboratory investigation of the merits of Ensol, but also as to its clinical value, an amount not to exceed $4,000. has been made available as from January first, to permit of a continuance of the Foundation's present programme.

The amount is in keeping with what was suggested as being sufficient to carry on the activities of the Foundation for one month. It is not the present intention of the Government to continue to pay this grant beyond that date noted; that is, the grant is limited to $4,000.
Yours very truly,
(signed) Harold J. Kirby
Minister of Health.

At my interview on November 30th with the Minister of Health, the advisability of any further attempts to procure a license from Ottawa either by the Foundation or the Ontario Government was discussed. It was the opinion of the Minister that maintenance of the Hendry-Connell Research Foundation as a research institution was essential from the Government's point of view since if it became necessary that the Foundation should receive aid from the Government this could only be done on a research basis. I stated to the Minister that as far as I was personally concerned although I had a very substantial personal interest in both the American and Canadian CAPCO organizations and that at the time these companies were formed it seemed the best policy to pursue, I now felt that it was essential that I should relinquish my holdings in these companies. This I am quite prepared to do. I also expressed the view that it would be best for the problem, and all concerned that no Director or Directors of the Foundation should in future in any way be associated with a commercialization programme. I also expressed the view that ultimate distribution to the public would best be done by any of the larger established pharmaceutical houses under license from the Foundation. If such a condition existed it would enable the Government, through its close association with the Foundation, to exercise a certain amount of control over distribution and price to the public. This is but fair in consideration of what the Government of Ontario has already done and what they have planned to do in the future. I left the Minister with the understanding that I would place this matter before Mr. Connolly as soon as possible since I expected to have an opportunity to see him in Montreal in the near future.

H. C. Connell
President

CHAPTER 9

1939-1945

It should be realized that it was a constant struggle and burden for Dr. Connell to finance the Hendry-Connell Research Foundation, oversee the expanding production of Ensol and deal with the new requests for the product constantly being received. The grants and other financial assistance received still did not cover all expenses. As well, it was necessary to continue with the research to improve Ensol and production methods. Hendry never lost sight of his avowed intention to provide Ensol at no charge, including delivery costs.

It was in mid 1939 that he began requesting assistance from the Ontario Government through the Minister of Health. The Foundation was eventually granted a monthly allowance of $3,000 until September 1942. This grant was to assist in the work of the Foundation in producing Ensol and making it available free of charge to physicians for use in the treatment of their cancer patients who were residents of and within the Province of Ontario. The source for this amount seems to have come from two different commissions or departments and was the subject of many letters requesting receipt of the cheque for $3,000, due that month and often for the previous month.

The problems caused by the Second World War were yet another obstacle the Hendry-Connell Research Foundation had to overcome during the next six years of conflict. The lack of experienced help and skilled technicians was an immediate and ongoing problem. The lack of funds was always present and there was competition throughout the country for qualified personnel. One of the Foundation's most experienced and qualified technicians left for a better paying job in Vancouver without a day's notice in 1941. Canada was now out of the

Depression and was in the middle of a boom with many wartime short-ages.

The following correspondence from Hendry Connell to two different Ontario Ministers of Health during 1943 will illustrate the problems constantly faced in the administration of the Foundation, apart from overseeing and being responsible for the production and research. Telegram sent via Canadian Pacific Telegraphs

Honourable H.J. Kirby,
March 15th, 1943
Minister of Health,
Parliament Buildings
Toronto, Ontario
Absolutely essential temporary financial assistance be sent before Friday this week STOP no wish to precipitate issue realizing your difficulties STOP if possible please give this your immediate attention.
H.C. Connell MD

Letter sent the same day as telegram

Honourable H.J. Kirby,
March 15th, 1943
Minister of Health
Parliament Buildings
Toronto, Ontario.

Dear Mr. Kirby:
This is to confirm and further explain my wire of even date.

I have no wish to hurry negotiations with the Department, but I have now no alternative. I am very grateful for all that has been done to assist me in this arduous task. In the hope that funds would have been received before this time from a private source, I have hesitated to request the Government for further aid. However, the funds which have been promised have not as yet been forthcoming and in the meantime it has been my personal duty to finance the work.

I have reached the end of my personal resources. I have had no remuneration for my services since October last, nor have some of the others of my staff. We have continued to supply treatment, free of charge, to several hundred cases having sent out since July last,

36,310 cc's postage paid to physicians throughout the country. This must cease since I cannot continue to carry the load. Requests continue to come in for further supplies daily in an ever widening field. I feel a grave responsibility toward the patients who are at present on treatment and do not, under any circumstances, wish to have any of them applying to you for further assistance. In the past such advances by patients to you have not been made with my knowledge or consent. I am sure that this has made it appear that we were trying to force the Government to do something for us. Let me assure you, Mr. Kirby that this is not the case. I feel, and have always felt, that such action on our part would not enhance the dignity of our work. The last report made to you by the Ontario Commission for the Investigation of Cancer remedies in which they stated that in their opinion this work should be continued and that this material should be used along with surgery and X-radiation in the treatment of malignancy, has been sufficient stimulus to me to do all in my power to keep sending the material to those who request it.

I am solely interested in the ethical conduct of the work and the furtherance of research since I am completely convinced of the importance of what has already been done, and that more concentrated effort, under less difficult conditions, will yield reward far beyond the value of the money expended.

It is, therefore, with all due respect and consideration to the difficulties which I know must fall to your lot that, I make this conscientious appeal for immediate assistance.
Yours sincerely

H.C. Connell

H.C. Connell, MD
HCC:AP

The following letter sent to the Minister of Health six months later continues to express the same problems and concerns which had been present throughout the entire life of the research project. That Hendry persevered in such adverse conditions can only show his belief that the treatment and control of cancer could be achieved. His determination, dedication and devotion to this work has yet to be acknowledged.

A letter to the new Minister follows,*

Personal
October 30th, 1943
Dr. R.P. Vivian,
Minister of Health,
Parliament Buildings,
Toronto, Ontario.

Dear Doctor Vivian:
The enclosed letter speaks for itself. I send it to you in an
absolutely confidential and impersonal manner. I receive such
letters all too frequently, but they stimulate me to further effort.
Perhaps it is a good thing that I get them even though they put me
'on the spot'.

We have underway and outlined for the near future, a programme which should result in considerable advance in our
present knowledge of this problem. When you said to me, "you
have two problems, one cancer research, and the other money"
you summed up my predicament precisely.

I am very thankful for all that has been done and is being done,
but without security for the continuance of the financial support, I
am constantly worried. I, therefore, hope that before long, you will
find it possible to discuss my difficulties with the other members
of your Government who may be in authority to make decisions.
At all times I am at your service and will be very happy to present
any information which might be required.

Please treat this letter as definitely personal and confidential. I
send it to you with sincerity and entirely devoid of personal interest, so that you may be aware of the size, scope and present need
for solution of the problem with which I have to deal.
Yours sincerely,

H.C. Connell

H.C. Connell, MD
HCC:AP

* The enclosed letter referred to is not available. The reader is left to his own
conclusion. The political changes of Ministers of Health didn't necessarily help in the
transfer of information regarding the grant money.

CHAPTER **10**

The two bulletins, No. 2 dated January, 1937 and Bulletin No. 3 dated March, 1938, both contain many case histories. Despite the large numbers, however, the time period only covered a few years. By 1946 the reports from those physicians attending cancer patients and administering Ensol continued to increase and to contain more useful information, adding eight more years of experience. It was case histories like this hand-written report that must have kept Hendry on an even keel during those past seven years. Each mail delivery brought similar letters.

This hand-written letter from Dr. W.B.P., MD of Montezuma, Iowa consists of eight pages, covering four case histories all written the same day, November 25th, 1946.

RG-white male age, 72 yrs
In the summer of 1939 this man noticed a pimple or sore upon his penis. He did nothing but the lesion enlarged and grew. He started using salve upon it but to no avail. In about 6 mo. he noticed swelling in his right groin. He went to his local doctor, W.B.C., MD of Io. & he told him it looked bad and might be a cancer. The doctor sent him as a private case to Dr. N.A. head of the Urology Dept. St. Univ. of Iowa, Iowa City, Iowa. He told him it was a cancer took a piece of it for a frozen section and the Path. Dept. confirmed the diagnosis. The inguinal lymph glands on the right side were resected and he was given an X-ray treatment. He was sent home and in a few months developed pain in his back (spine). He went to Mercy Hosp, at Oskaloosa because it was closer to his house. The Mercy Hosp. X-rayed his back and told his family the cancer had settled in his spine, that they could do nothing but

would give him some deep X-ray therapy which might be palla-
tive. He took quite a few of these but gradually got worse. Finally
they told his family & his doctor that they could not give any more
X-ray treatments, for him to go home that his local doctor would
take care of him. He was taking morphine for his pain. He heard I
was giving my brother, Dr. W.R.P. a cancer serum & he was getting better. His wife & son brought him up to see me May 10-
1940. He was emaciated, very weak, constant pain had lost considerable weight. The lesion in the rt groin had broken down and the
odor was terrific. The pus & discharge had run clear to his ankle
and his leg was excoriated its length where the discharge had run.
I told him he was too far gone & advised against Ensol but he
insisted upon taking it. He was started out that day upon 1/2 cc &
each day the Ensol was increased 1/4 cc until he got to 10 cc &
that daily dose was maintained. In 2 wks his draining sluffing
groin lesion was healed smooth. He took daily shots for about 5
mo. then every other day for 1 mo, then twice a wk for 1 mo. He
then quit. He gained back all his weight & went back to farming.
He is still living, has retired & moved. He has never had any sign
of a reoccurrance. He was in my office about 1 mo. ago.
W.B.P., MD
Nov. 25, 1946

C.Z.-white male, age 50
In Oct., 1942 Mr. Z consulted me for loss of wt. Weakness gas &
pain in his stomach. His normal wt. was 220. His weight when he
consulted me was 160 lbs. His stomach had bothered him for 6 or
8 mo & he was now upon a milk and eggnog diet because most
every thing else hurt his stomach. He was a telephone repair &
linesman working for the local telephone Co. here. I advised an
X-ray but couldn't get off work he said. I told him he probably had
a ca or ulcer. I insisted upon an X-ray, offered to take him 50 mi
distance for nothing, but he would have to pay for his own X-ray.
In 2 wks he made up his mind & I took him to Dr. S.F.S. roentge-
nologist who diagnosed it for advanced ca of stomach. Mr. Z then
made arrangement to enter the State Univ. Hosp. of Iowa City as
an indigent case. After gastroscopic X-ray etc exam they resected
60% of his stomach, the operation taking 5-1/2 hr. I watched the

operation & they told me there, 18 to 24 mo. was his limit, that it was impossible to remove all the mesenteric glands that drained the ca. A frozen section there confirmed the diagnosis. He was operated upon the first week in Dec 1944. In about 1 mo he came home from the hosp. & started taking Ensol. A friend & neighbor who is a trained nurse gives it to him. His 2 yrs is practically up now. He works every da as a general telephone repair man. Present wt. 180 a gain of 20 lbs. strength good, no symptoms & no complaints except he has to eat 5 or 6 times a day as the limit of his stomach capacity is about one pint. He has taken for about 22 mo. 5 cc of Ensol every other day. Today an order goes in for more Ensol for him. He has done better than I anticipated, what the ultimate outcome will be only time can tell.

W.B.P., MD

Nov. 25, 1946

Dr. W.R.P., white male age 40

The above patient my brother drove to Davenport Ia 150 mi. to consult me in Sept 1939. He was jaundiced very weak and had lost from 150 to 130 lbs in wt. in 2 mos. I had seen him 2 months prior and he looked OK and did not complain at that time. He gave a history of gradual progressive weakness over a 6 mo and several attacks of diarrhoea. He had fever 15,000 white count, urine negative except for considerable bile. He was tender and some rigidity over McBurneys point and that I could feel a mass there. I made the arrangements for him to the St. University of Iowa Hospital the next morn. That night he had another attack of diarrohea. The next da he entered the hospital as a private case. They left him under observation for several da and then did a barium enema.

Halfway up the ascending colon he had a block and barium couldn't go thru. They planned a two stage bowel resection but when they got in there they found the liver full of metastasic nodules. Some mesenteric lymph glands were removed for section an ileocolostomy done and he was closed up. The section from mesenteric nodes showed a rapid growing adeno ca. He developed a post operative pneumonia, was given sulphapyradine and finally recovered. Dr. F.P. head of surgery dept gave him 2 mo. to live under no circumstances over 6 mo. as he said he was far advanced. He was brought to his home about Oct. 20 '39 and started upon Ensol 1/2 cc and increased 1/4 cc every da until up to 20 cc then held on 20 cc daily. Soon after coming home his side swelled up and 8 oz. of pus was removed and drain tubes put in. It drained for about 30 da. In 2 mo he was able to be up and around but weighed only 112 lbs. I then moved to take care of him as my father a physician and surgeon but retired was afraid to give him the Ensol as he got too many reactions.

My brother continued to improve and by mid summer of 1940 weighed 145, went back to part time veterinary work and took several weekend fishing trips into Minnesota 200 mi distance. He ate good, slept good looked good except at times he would jaundice up. His strength was moderate. That summer I took him back up to see Dr. P. and he was astonished to see him even alive. In Oct. 1940 one yr. after his operation he took Scarlet Fever and had a severe case of it. He recovered and in Nov. 1940 went pheasant hunting with me 200 mi. distance and walked me down.

However in Dec 1940 he started to complain of back ache if he walked much. This got gradually worse and by Feb. 1941 he started losing weight. The Ensol never seemed to help him after he had Scarlet Fever. By July 41 he was bed fast and died middle of Aug. 41 weight 60 lbs. post mortem confirmed what an X-ray showed in his spine 8 mo. previous. His liver was mostly ca tissue his intestines matted together and mesenteric lymph glands involved. About 2 quarts pus in pelvic cavity.

W.B.P., MD

Nov. 25, 1946

Mrs. R.P.O. age 56

This report has to do with another of my immediate family, my sister. In Aug 1939, while I was visiting over the wk end at her house she mentioned she had been having spotting for about a yr & of late was having mild pains which shot around in her pelvis now & then. She had lost no weight & strength was normal. Her menopause was six yrs ago. I made arrangement & took her as a private patient to Dr. J.H.R. of Gyn. Dept. St. Univ. of Iowa Hosp. A D&C was done and a frozen section showed adeno ca of fundus.

Radium was inserted & in a few da. she came home. She returned in one mo. for a panhysterectomy. In the fall of 1939 I started her upon Ensol. About 5cc was about as high as she could get without reactions. She continued this dosage daily for about 2 yr. then every other day for about a yr. then once or twice a wk for a yr. She was examined several times by Dr. R. but at no time could he find any sign of a reoccurrance. For about 18 mo. after her operation she bloated & had considerable trouble with gas in the bowels. As time went on that disappeared. Today she is living & in good health. Her prognosis at the time of her operation was given by Dr. R. as a 50-50 chance for a 5 yr. cure. What she would have done without the Ensol I don't know. I think it should have part of the credit as I have seen or heard of very few ca of fundus of uterus with symptoms of one year standing, the patient being alive & well 7 yrs after any operation, radium, X-ray or combination.
W.B.P. M.D
Nov. 25, 1946

During the years from 1935 to 1945 Dr. Connell submitted and had published many papers in the *Journal* of the Canadian Medical Association.

We now learn from correspondence and documents that the Federal Department of Health recognized the work of the Hendry-Connell Research Foundation and granted a licence for the manufacture and sale of the Ensol material in Canada in March, 1946. Literature was produced and circulated to physicians, hospitals and clinics in Canada only. It was sold in Canada by the unit at $20.00 for six vials of 10 cc each. In the United States however, because no application had been made for a licence, the Foundation continued to supply Ensol free of charge to those patients and doctors who requested it. However, the Foundation was now free to accept grants or donations from US users toward research, if any cheques were so designated. There were many users in the United States but the opportunity now to accept donations for research was not the bonanza it might appear, as such donations were few. It was necessary to find more skilled staff, sources for tissue and various packaging supplies. Shortages in most categories were still a problem in this post-war period. Costs and expenses continued to outpace revenue by a considerable margin.

Perhaps one bright light during the war years was the fact that the Kingston General Hospital did not insist that the laboratory building on their property be removed as the original agreement required.

Nevertheless the building was dismantled in 1947 and the laboratory moved to a basement location in St. Mary's of the Lake Hospital on King Street West, and was again moved to a location on Division Street in 1949, where it remained until 1951.

Despite the use of Ensol in many locations, the US and elsewhere, there was lack of marketing and distribution experience within the Hendry-Connell Research Foundation; still, a number of attempts were made to have distributors handle the product.

Some of the distributors were:

SMALLWOOD PHARMACEUTICALS LIMITED of Orangeville, Ontario, appears to be the first company to sign an agreement in 1945. However, the Foundation soon cancelled it and Smallwood returned 5000 vials in early May, 1946. This agreement was short lived. There is no record of the reason for this abrupt cancellation, but it is assumed that the normal discount of 40% due a distributing agency deducted from the twenty dollar price set by the Foundation did not nearly cover the cost of production.

HENDRY-CONNELL RESEARCH FOUNDATION Kingston, Ontario. From records and correspondence it would seem that the Foundation again made every effort to distribute and sell Ensol where possible. It was in the spring of 1946 that a skilled and qualified bacteriologist, Dr. R. Glasser, was employed to produce Ensol and also to carry out the tests as required by the various government regulations (principally sterility and non-pyrogenic tests) to ensure the product was safe to administer to cancer patients.

Again this attempt to produce sufficient revenue for the operation was not successful but probably allowed the Foundation to keep more of the twenty dollar unit charge.

CO-DRUGS LIMITED, Kingston, Ontario, was formed in 1949 to generate revenue for Hendry's further research efforts. The products consisted of such items as aspirin, aspirin-codeine, laxatives and ammoniated dentifrices. Co-Drugs was also to be a distributor for the US Vitamin Corporation. These products were produced and/or repackaged at the Division Street location. However, the sale and distribution in an increasingly competitive market resulted in this venture not being a success and all operations were discontinued in 1951.

THE J.F. HARTZ CO. LIMITED Toronto, Ontario. There is an existing letter dated 9th November, 1949, from a Mr. A.A.S., vice president, agreeing to carry a stock of Ensol for distribution to physicians and hospitals, at a price to be set by the Foundation, Hartz's remuneration to be a discount of 40% from such a price. Hartz's salesmen were to take out literature to be supplied and make it thoroughly known that they could supply Ensol promptly on request. They were also to attend a lecture on the product to be given by Dr. Hendry Connell. There is no evidence that there was any further association with this company. It is assumed that the proposed normal discount may have been the stumbling block if the Foundation was trying to maintain the price of twenty dollars per unit when supplying Ensol directly. Distribution through a wholesaler would have necessitated a dramatic increase in the unit price that would have been contrary to Hendry's intention. (In today's world, the price would have been increased).

FELIX N. RODRIGUEZ Ciudad Trujillo, Dominican Republic. This distributor of pharmaceutical products received samples in Aug. and Oct. of 1948 and two shipments of 100 vials each Aug. and Sept. 1949. No further record of any further transactions exist.

BAXTER LABORATORIES INC. Morton Grove, Chicago, Illinois. Association with this firm is the last recorded attempt to continue the production and further research on Ensol by Dr. Hendry C. Connell and the Foundation. Hendry wrote to Baxter requesting their help and hoping they would be interested enough to take over his work. On November 21, 1951, employment contracts dated November 1, 1951 were received in Kingston for Hendry and Dr. Lloyd Munro. These two contracts covered the two doctors, each to be retained as scientific consultants for a retainer of $500.00 per month for two years. It was agreed that the contracts could not be terminated prior to November 1, 1953. Baxter then sent Dr. R.M. Petersen, a biochemist who was to be in charge of a lab set up on the second floor of the Golden Lion Block, Wellington St. in Kingston, Ontario. This was for production of Ensol (Renamed U-10 by Baxter) and further research, with Drs. Connell and Munro consulting and advising on the operation.

There was a considerable supply of U-10 returned to the Baxter labs in Morton Grove at the end of this period.

Unfortunately some time after his return to Baxter (it was learned in 1968) Dr. Petersen became ill, was "confined to an institution" and never returned to work. Nothing seems to have happened because he was the only one with any knowledge of the procedures. After over forty years, investigation has not uncovered the existence of Dr. R.M. Petersen's papers.

During this period Dr. Connell returned to his medical practice in his original office on King street. Disqualifying himself from operating after so many years, he applied for a refresher course in Rochester, New York, which never materialized because there were not enough applicants. But he maintained a very busy practice until 1963, with many grateful patients. (In 1958 Hendry was hospitalized for a short duration because of a stroke.)

Hendry was of course still receiving correspondence and inquiries about Ensol and its supply. It would appear that for supply, all requests were referred to Baxter and when they made the decision to destroy their existing supply of U-10 and not market it, the supply stopped. It is not known why Baxter did not continue with production but there could have been many reasons for a large firm to make such a decision. Patent infringements might have been one reason, marketing another, or yet a third might have been a decision to keep it off the market. Although the volume of production was large and expanding from the Foundation's view, to go into production might not have been profitable enough to satisfy Baxter's investors. Pharmaceutical companies like most other companies, must be profitable and are not charitable institutions. Correspondence from Baxter seemed to end.

CHAPTER **11**

DR. CALVIN HENDRY CAMERON CONNELL'S
LAST DAYS

In 1958, Hendry was admitted to Kingston General Hospital for a myocardial infarction involving the inferior wall of the left ventrical and acute congestive heart failure.

In 1961 he was admitted for acute bronchitis and arteriosclerotic heart disease and in July, 1963, for congestive heart failure and in August for severe nose bleed. While in hospital he developed shortness of breath. A chest X-ray revealed pulmonary congestion. He improved with treatment. He was also having severe back pain periodically. On testing there was no evidence of aneurysm or gastro-intestinal lesion, only diverticulosis in the sigmoid colon.

No one reports of the stress this man had been under for many years regarding his work or the birth of another child in his late forties, of the care of his ill wife and his aging father, or of losing his first son, who was confined to an institution because of a lobotomy during the war years.

During the one month of Hendry's hospitalization he continuously complained of severe abdominal pain, which required large doses of narcotics. Hendry himself, and one of his medical colleagues, Dr. George Myer, used to sit up late in the night and discuss his work and his condition.

(At this time he also often spoke of Baxter and asked if anyone had had any correspondence relating to his work. He was not aware of Dr. Petersen's confinement on his return to the Baxter Laboratory, Morton Grove.)

He and his colleague suspected Hendry had cancer for some time before the physicians in charge finally ordered a laparotomy and, in the middle of the night on November 8th, 1963, the operation revealed a large tumour mass involving the body tail and head of the pancreas.

Before the operation Hendry said that if it was cancer he did not want to have 'cobalt bomb' treatment. He wanted to use his enzyme solution, Ensol, only (this request was ignored or he changed his mind under pressure, and on November 12th and 13th, he was treated with cobalt, a radiation therapy replacing radium and radon) which would kill the cancerous cells. Morphine and then Schlesenger's solution were administered for pain. The clinical course was a slow progression downhill. He was in and out of congestive heart failure on many occasions. His ECG showed sinus rhythm with first degree heart bloc and old inferior wall myocardial infarction.

Over the years from the first production of Ensol, Hendry had always been the first to be inoculated with a new batch of the enzyme solution. He would take several cc's to be sure the serum was safe. It was ironic to find he had cancer. The notes on the dosages of Ensol he was administered following the detection of his cancerous condition show how the strength of the Schlesenger's solution he received for pain slowly regressed. During his last few days he showed signs of congestive heart failure and he died at 4:45 p.m. on January 30, 1964.

Dr. Forde Connell, in whose care Hendry was, said: "No one should have had so little pain having that amount of cancerous disease. There must have been something in Ensol after all. Hendry died a brave and sad man!"

After writing about my father, we now understand his intense feeling about this quotation which he had hanging on his wall wherever he went and quoted to us year after year.

*And I said to the man who stood at the gate of the year: "Give me
a light that I may tread safely into the unknown." And he
replied: "Go out into the darkness and put your hand into the
hand of God. That shall be to you better than the known way."
So I went forth and finding the Hand of God, trod gladly into the
night. And he led me towards the hills and the breaking of day in
the lone East.*

The Kingston Whig-Standard published an interview with Dr. Connell by Star Staff Correspondent Roy Greenaway in the mid 50's. Reprinted with permission of The Toronto Star Syndicate.

BLOW TO WORK ON CANCER SEEN IN BOGOMOLETZ DEATH

BY ROY GREENAWAY
Star Staff Correspondent

Kingston, July 22. To Dr. H.C. Connell, the only man in Canada with first hand knowledge of the work of Dr. Alexander Bogomoletz, death of the Russian scientist Saturday came as a shock.

"Biologic research in cancer has suffered a severe blow," the Kingston scientist said today. "Dr. Bogomoletz' efforts were always directed toward the betterment of mankind. He worked in a field of science which never has received the degree of support so blithely given the advancement of new and more deadly methods of destruction. For this reason, if for no other, his name for all time to come will take its place beside the truly great in the history of the world."

"Dr. Bogomoletz pioneered in the field of the clinical application of a biologic theory in the treatment of cancer and other diseases resistant to modern methods of treatment," continued Dr. Connell. "His work has been criticized freely and not too generously at times, both in the med-

ical and lay press, before its real significance was fully appreciated. Recently an investigation under way at the department of anatomy and preventive medicine, University of Texas, concerning the growing inhibitory and reticular stimulating effects of his A.R.C.S. (anti-reticular cytoxic serum) have confirmed his results."

To Dr. Connell, discoverer of the new tumor antigen Ensol, there is nothing fantastic about the assertion that the use of the Bogomoletz A.C.S. (anti-reticular cytoxic serum) may lead to a longer life.

First-Hand Knowledge
The only man in Canada to have first-hand knowledge of the A.C.S. serum, Dr. Connell has been making and using the serum on experimental animals as a check to some of his work in cancer research since May 1, 1944.

"Dr. Bogomoletz did not make the statement that the use of his serum will make one live to the age of 150," explained Dr. Connell. What he really said was that the natural span of human life should be approximate-

ly 150 years, and that one's age is dependent upon the state of the connective tissue elements of the body which can be stimulated by an A.C.S. serum helping to defer natural degeneration."

"If, and I understand it is, the Bogomoletz serum is being widely used in Russia today, it is reasonable to assume that a certain percentage of the population so treated will not age as rapidly as they would have done without this stimulation," he continued. "The treatment would have to be given two or three times a year to be effective and to prove its longevity effects in humans. A long period of time and observation would be necessary. Prof. Bogomoletz emphasized that it should not be given to people with heart lesion."

Vital Factor
Dr. Connell said that while the Bogomoletz serum is not in any sense a specific agent for cancer, its use might eventually lessen the incidence of cancer, since the A.C.S. serum stimulates the reticular tissues of the body whose function it is to combat disease, and in the body's efforts to control

133

cancer, stimulation of the connective tissue elements is an important factor.

The recticulo-endothelial tissue of the body includes all body cells known to have a hand in the protective mechanism against disease. These cells are found principally in the spleen, certain cells of the liver, the large cells lining the blood vessels, some parts of the lymphatic tissues, the bone marrow and so forth.

"The Bogomoletz serum stimulates the connective tissue side of the reticulo-endothelial system helping in the production of clasmatocytes, fibroblasts and other large protective cells," said Dr. Connell. "It also, to use Bogomoletz own words, 'Sets fire to the haemato-paryenchymal barrier,' the reservoir which he believes to exist in the intra cellular spaces containing the materials from which the body cells themselves receive their nourishment."

Ever since 1936, as Dr. Connell's publications attested, he believed the reticulo-endothelial system plays an important part in recovery from cancer. It was obvious from work done in his laboratories at Kingston and at other laboratories in the United States and elsewhere, that in cancer patients this system of cells was damaged.

Okayed by Commission

"The natural effort of the body to fight the disease by producing antibodies against the cancer cells is resident in this tissue," explained Dr. Connell. He said that Ensol has produced a substance which stimulates the production of tumor tissue antibodies. This work was checked by an independent Ontario government research laboratory set up at Kingston and the Ontario cancer commission stated Ensol had a beneficial effect in the treatment of malignant disease. This product is now manufactured in quantity for general use under federal license. Its price was fixed by the Wartime prices and trade board and it is now available to physicians, hospitals and clinics.

Since the Connell antigen was a specific stimulating antigen calculated to induce the reticulo endothelial system to produce antibodies against malignant growth it was valuable to Dr. Connell to obtain the Bogomoletz serum to check some of his work.

"Results have been spectacular," said Dr. Connell. "Experiments with cancer bearing animals showed that when they were stimulated with the Bogomoletz serum the speed of tumor growth was significantly depressed, even though this serum had nothing to do with cancer specifically but was a general reticular stimulant. On the other hand, if the reticular system were blocked the speed of tumor growth was very markedly increased, and the spread of the disease in the blocked animal was such that in all animals the group so treated were dead in a nine-day period. Animals without treatment lived approximately 36 days.

Prove Fundamentals

"The work of Bogomoletz," said Dr. Connell, "therefore is of great value as it helped to prove some of the fundamental principles by which the body tries to overcome disease and confirmed the importance of the reticulo-endothelial system in any study of the cancer problem."

Another important fact in the latest research of Dr. Connell and his associates which will be reported through the usual medical channels in the near future is that it appears that the malignant cells themselves throw out substances into the blood stream of the patient in sufficient quantities to so damage the reticulo-endothelial cells as to render them incapable of producing antibodies even when stimulated-in other words the cancer itself produces a particular type of reticular block.

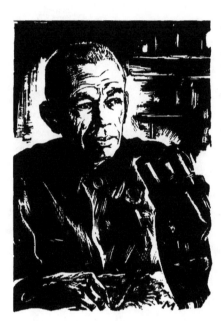

Alexander A. Bogomoletz

A scientist of vision and a brilliant executive, Bogomoletz did pioneer work in the field of blood transfusions and from this beginning there developed a vast network of blood banks. In 1930 he moved from Moscow to Kiev to become the founder and Director of the Kiev Institute of Experimental Biology and Pathology.

The day after the Nazi attack, June 23, 1941, a cable from Moscow announced to the world, that the life-prolonging serum Bogomoletz sought had been perfected. The war curtailed further experiments on longevity and his institute's activities were directed to producing enough serum to meet the needs of the battlefield. It was with this scientist's experimental work that H.C. Connell became so familiar.

135

Report on Dupont Papers recovered from

Hagley Museum and Library

Wilmington , Delaware

assisted by
Marjorie G. McNinch
Manuscripts & Archives department

October 2 0 0 3

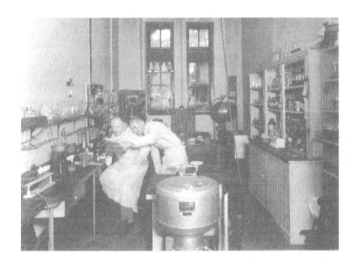

SUPPLEMENT TO THE STORY OF ENSOL

Acquiring our so-called "Dupont Papers ' has added a great deal of information , which unfortunately was not known to exist or to be available to the authors of "Enzyme Solution --the Story of Ensol" at the time of publication in the year 2001.

The researcher was discouraged when further information was not forthcoming from the Franklin Institute in Philadelphia regarding the existence or history of the Biochemical Research Foundation, even though that organization was founded as an adjunct of the Franklin Institute December 1st ,1935. This date is six months after the announcement of Hendry Connell's invention of Ensol in July,1935.

A first review of this collection of letters has immediately revealed to the authors how little of the full story about Ensol they ever did uncover from those records available to them in Kingston. Somehow and somewhere most copies of letters and replies between Dr. Mcdonald of Philadelphia, Dr. Connell of Kingston and their benefactor Mr. Irenee Dupont of Wilmington Delaware, are missing from any known Kingston collection of records. This new collection tells so much about those persons whose aim was the successful treatment and cure of cancer, through the production and distribution of the invention of Dr. Hendry C Connell of Kingston , Ontario.

The serious difference of opinions and attitudes that developed not long after an agreement was signed between the Franklin Institute Research Laboratory in Philadelphia and the Hendry-Connell Research Foundation in Kingston late fall 1935, are recorded in detail in these very frank exchanges of correspondence between the principals. Mr Dupont is most patient and of course, most generous in all the proceedings and references. His unusual method of donating funds in addition to his regular grants to both the Biochemical Research Foundation in the US and the Hendry-Connell Research Foundation in Canada was indeed remarkable. Mr. Dupont would often send an endorsed stock certificate with his advice regarding the present cash value or the expected future value of a stock like Phillips Petroleum. In all his correspondence he was very patient and understanding of the pressures experienced and views expressed in the progress .
With this new information from the Hagley Museum and Library our story immediately becomes international in its scope, interest and as well, presents absorbing moments.

In 1927 Irenee Dupont was introduced to Dr Ellice Mcdonald who had for some years been interested in the chemotherapy approach to the problem of cancer, believing "that surgery and x-ray were fast approaching their limits in the treatment of cancer". Mr Dupont became much interested in Dr. Mcdonald's ideas and in November 1927 provided the first grant to help him conduct independent research at the University of Pennsylvania. This regular grant of money was earmarked for Dr. Macdonald's independent research. This arrangement continued for eight years. On December 1 1935 the Biochemical Research Foundation with Dr. Mcdonald as director was founded as an adjunct of the Franklin Institute in Philadelphia. This foundation was always supported entirely by Mr. Dupont with the Franklin Institute acting as trustee only.

Meanwhile across the border, in Kingston, Ontario Dr. Hendry Connell who in 1929 was appointed assistant professor in the Faculty of Medicine of Queen's University teaching the treatment of diseases in his specialties of the ear, eye, nose and throat, by 1930 had begun research to find a method of dissolving the cataract of the eye. It was a private research conducted on a part time basis and carried out after hours. His only assistant was a young laboratory technician

3

who was associated with the Department of Bacteriology at Queen's University. Hendry financed his research from his own funds apart from a $500.00 grant from the National Research Council of Canada in Ottawa. Over five years this work led to the discovery of a substance having a specific action upon carcinoma tisssue. In 1935 after many tests and carefully kept case histories, an announcement was published in the Canadian Medical Association Journal of the discovery of this 'enzyme' solution cancer treatment named Ensol. (enzyme in solution). As we read later the active principle in bacterial filtrates they had produced was not an ENZYME but an ANTIGEN

By coincidence , the announcement of the discovery of the treatment by Ensol in the summer of 1935 in Kingston and the formation in December 1935, of the Biochemical Research Foundation as an adjunct of the Franklin Institute of Philadelphia, brought together two researchers with identical aims and views at the same time in history.

It was in November 1935 that Dr. Ellice Mcdonald, still working at the University of Pennsylvania, invited Hendry Connell and his assistant there for a discussion of their plans. Dr. Mcdonald reported in a letter to Mr. Irenee Dupont that he was very impressed with the 'Canadian'. His letter also mentions the decision to call the product 'Rex' in his laboratory and of his concern of any news getting into the papers. at this early stage of the aggreement made between Connell and Mcdonald. Mcdonald does seem to indicate to Mr, Dupont and that he has taken command.

Other letters determine that the issuing of stock in the Kingston Foundation to various individuals is merely intended to qualify that individual as a director of the Hendry-Connell Research Foundation only, and have no value.

At this early date into the agreement, there is a discussion regarding patents. The Hendry-Connell Research Foundation states they are willing to have Mr Dupont and his legal department look after all patent applications. Mr Arthur Connolly (Dupont lawyer) enters the story and has an important role and keen interest in "protecting Hendry's invention and the future life and value of Ensol."

Dr. Mcdonald visited Kingston December 6th and 7th ,1935 and on his return wrote to Mr Dupont that he had talked to the Dept. Minister of Health." This is presumed to mean the Deputy Minister .
Mcdonald also thinks a visit to Mackenzie King , Prime Minister, an old friend of his, would be helpful . Dr Mcdonald was a graduate of Mcgill.. He also appears to be a namedropper in his letters to Dupont.

From this and other letters, the reviewer is beginning to form the opinion that Dr. Mcdonald is very concerned, even at this early date, that Mr. Dupont not be allowed too close to Hendry Connell and that all contact be through Mcdonald only. It is as though he feels threatened, that his close contact and financing over the last eight years is in jeopardy, and that Mr.Dupont must not be allowed to form his own opinion or understanding of the facts. It is already evident that the close exchange and deliberation with Dr. Mcdonald is declining. Many of Mcdonald's letters are now becoming lengthy and are somewhat ponderous. He is a graduate of Mcgill University but we have yet to determine his nationality. At this time, his age would be 59 or 60 years of age. Hendry Connell is about 40 at this time.

As 1936 grows longer the activity at the Hendry-Connell Research Foundation seems more intense and certainly more meaningful, because of the new lab and $50,000.00 grant from Dupont. Arthur Connolly confirmed to Dr. J.C Connell, (Hendry's father) that Irenee Dupont has a "deep interest" in this cancer work which prompted Dr J.C. to write to Mr.Dupont offering to send a comprehensive review of the work of the Foundation
On May 30th 1936 Dupont writes of a "go"* for the Kingston Foundation. he writes "needless to say I am very much reassured and more optimistic than ever that your foundation should get it. It is perfectly evident that every effort should be made to get Ensol into volume production as soon as possible" Dupont suggests showing his company doctors the report. Dr. J.C.. writes back of his reservations because of the pictures of patients which are not for publication and "medical men object to apparent exploitation".

* note: The "go" in this letter refers to Mr. Dupont's suggestion that he send an additional $50,000.00 to the Hendry-Connell Research Foundation in Kingston to assist them in organizing a production line to manufacture Ensol for distribution and to relieve that laboratory for research exclusively. This was considered somewhat premature.

June, 1936 Harry B. Muir , editor of the Kingston Whig Standard, spoke to the Kiwanis Club of London Ontario. He spoke of the progress and success of Hendry Connell's Research work in the treatment of cancer.. He chose this subject when he was invited and honoured to preside at this meeting as a Past President of this club. he was reported as telling of the many many inquiries he had had on this subject from his friends and acquaintances in the London area.

This same summer, the general manager of Parke Davis Pharmaceutical Company was to meet in Kingston with all the directors of the two foundations "especially looking forward to the early general use of these preparations"

The next word of encouragement is through Dr. Neville Davis, in Australia who was an early supporter and who was treating cancer patients with Ensol with considerable success. He was receiving a regular supply of the product, shipped under constant refrigeration during passage. Due to Dr. Davis, the Australian Government was prepared to grant funds to further the production of the product Ensol.

The letters continue and one dated 23 rd July,1936 with a proposed agreement with Parke Davis and comments regarding the Australian interest.. Their government was evidently willing to pay $50,000.00 for a six month option and in the event that it was affirmatively exercised the option was to pay an annual lump sum plus 10% royalty.
This apparently was more than the Parke Davis offer and it was decided to up the anti to Parke Davis.

During the period of October 1936 into January 1937 Mr. Arthur Connolly was making every effort possible to provide and complete all the details necessary and required for the Connell US patent application.
Dr. Richard Street in Chicago to Dr. Mcdonald appears to be a report on the activity in operating his cancer clinic and of his impressions of a visit to the Kingston Foundation. It is certainly light hearted and with somewhat friendly comments. It is the only reference of any such clinic in Dupont's file of letters from Mcdonald.

The collection of letters, dated February and March of 1937, contains a number which identify some of the problems concerning various plans and ideas for the production of Ensol in quantity for distribution to those doctors requesting supplies. This demand for Ensol is increasing and the Kingston laboratory with it's limited capacity is falling behind in meeting this requirement. Again Mr.Dupont offers the money, through a letter to Connolly , to start up a company to manufacture Ensol to relieve the laboratories of this burden and concentrate on research. Mr. Dupont is most emphatic in this letter that he not receive any stock of such a company and that any such stock be in the hands of one or more of the Foundation's directors as trustees and any future profits be used for research. The tone if not the intent of this letter seems to indicate that Arthur Connolly come up with a plan acceptable to all concerned . Mr.Dupont seems very keen on what is going on in Kingston and is lacking enthusiatic reports from Mcdonald on activity in Philadelphia. not much in these files at any rate !

Back in April Mr. Dupont received a letter from Dr. Mcdonald dated 9th April ,1937 very critical of the Connells and Connolly and their relationship. also critical of the recent product runs of Ensol. Mcdonald seems to be starting a campaign to become more dominant on the board of directors by the appointment of two more acquaintances.
The reader should be reminded that Mr. Dupont had been providing Dr. Mcdonald with annual grants since 1927 to fund his independent cancer research while at the University of Pennsylvania teaching gynaecology. In the fall of 1935 Dupont footed the cost of the development of the Biochemical Research Foundation with The Franklin Institute as trustee and Mcdonald became director. At this same time Dupont became aware of the product Ensol discovered by Connell in Kingston and of the success in the clinical trials. Dupont was responsible for the agreement that was promptly made between

the Hendry -Connell Research Foundation and the Biochemical Research Foundation of Philadelphia. That autumn, he provided grants to both foundations so that research could continue with shared knowledge and close cooperation.

The agreement has now been in place only fifteen months when this letter of 9th April was written. Mcdonald seems determined to put the Kingston operation in a poor light as well as the work by Arthur Connolly of the legal office. He also places great confidence in statements by a Dr.Mundell who apparently contacted him after being dismissed from the position of cancer clinic head in the Kingston General Hospital for "his attitude and actions along with adverse information to patients, discouraging them from taking Ensol or following the policy that Ensol is supplied at no cost". One gets the impression from this and later letters that Mcdonald is quite determined to retain the position with Mr. Dupont that he has held for ten years as his medical counsellor on cancer research. It also appears that Dupont very much appreciates and admires the work done in Hendry Connell's laboratory and is anxious that it maintain and increase production of Ensol for distribution at no cost.

All of Mcdonald's letters appear to be composed with the expectation that Mr.Dupont will read them and be pleased how well things are going under Mcdonald's command. Mr Dupont does not seem deceived but is doing his utmost to promote the development and production of Ensol.
Mcdonald is writing lengthy letters to most everyone involved. This correspondence ends with Mr. Dupont's letter of 13th August 1937 to Hendry Connell asking that his suggestion to Mcdonald that the agreement be terminated, "be put in cold storage" until Mcdonald's return from a month's rest overseas. One wonders if that could have been Dupont's Cuban retreat.

The next letters in the file deal with separate developments.
On the 2nd August'37 Dupont is thanking Connolly for forwarding the congressional record of the Joint House Committee in Washington, on proposed cancer legislation to which H.C. Connell had been invited to attend and testify . This invitation was distinctive because he was the only doctor outside of the United States to be invited. Mr. Connolly was able to introduce into the records of the committee both bulletins of the Hendry-Connell Research Foundation and they are now officially filed as part of the record . Dupont wrote that he was "glad that Dr. Connell was given the attention that he so well deserves"
Dr. Connell wrote to Irenee Dupont in August 1937. This letter referred to his earlier one to Dr. Mcdonald about terminating the agreement which is copied in full in this file. This letter also keeps Mr. Dupont informed on the progress of work in Kingston. In July a total of 10 litres of Ensol was used in the laboratory or distributed. Hendry writes that his greatest problem is to get sufficient cancer tissue to produce enough Ensol to meet all requirements.

When last in Washington, he had arranged with the Surgeon -General that he be sent all the tissue available at the Walter Reed General Hospital. Surgeon-General Metcalfe was using Ensol on an important patient under his care in that hospital. In this rather lengthy letter Hendry encloses comments from the many letters or indeed, the letters themselves from physicians around the world. Many reports of success and always of relief from pain and reduction in the use of pain-killing morphine. **Recently , in the Kingston laboratory , they had discovered that the active principle in bacterial filtrates they had been producing was not an " enzyme but an antigen"** This discovery was important in that it held the promise of immunization or standardization, Confirmation by further tests would change the aspect of the research and consequently affect the patients. This letter ends with a suggestion to go down to see Connolly and if convenient to Mr. Dupont, to visit him and tell of these developments in detail and to consult on the proper course for the future.

The next letter to Mr. Irenee Dupont is again from Kingston containing a copy of the minutes of a meeting of the Hendry-Connell Research Foundation held 10th August, 1937.
The following is copied from the minutes.
Present H.C.Connell J.C.Connell
B.J.Holsgrove G.F.Mooers Sec.

The monthly report on patients was presented as follows

	July 1937
Admitted	9
Diagnosed as not "ca"	1
Examined and home for surgery	1
Left on own accord	1
No. of new cases	6
Total no. of Ensol treatments given in clinic for July	348
Total no. of cc'c for July	873.5 cc's
Total no. of patients treated in clinic for July	47
Last register no. for July	915
Total no. of cc's shipped outside clinic	6330 cc's

* No new physicians sent Ensol in July

No communications have been received from Dr. Mcdonald since the last meeting of the board of directors. Dr. Mcdonald has not visited the laboratory since June 25th, 1936. In view of his lack of interest I have written to him suggesting cancellation of the agreement by mutual consent on terms to be agreed upon.

On motion the meeting adjourned.
H.C.Connell, MD

Mr. Irenee Dupont writes to Dr. Mcdonald on 16th November 1937 transferring 200 shares of Christiana Securities Company. which he expects will take care of Mcdonald's budget for the year ending October 1939. From this contribution Mcdonald is instructed to send "forthwith" Dr. Connell's last payment of $25,000.00 under the contract. Mr. Dupont goes on to say that the possibility of a general financial collapse of the National economy could put an end to contributions by him toward Dr. Mcdonald's work..

There is an exchange of letters between Arthur Connolly and Dr Mcdonald regarding the patent application re: Connell Ser.137,931 on which Mcdonald now wants to change his affidavit. Connolly writes
" that I shall be very happy to do my best in order to withhold filing a copy of your affidavit dated March,19th,1936. I can well appreciate the fact that as this picture develops, allegations which originally appeared to be correct are now looked upon with some doubt and, on the other hand, allegations which might originally have been considered unsound, may now be free from objection."

In a letter to Mr.Dupont from the board of directors of the Hendry-Connell Research Foundation dated 27th January 1938 , he was advised that a resolution had been passed, thanking him for his generous support which made it possible to relieve the suffering and prolong the lives of some hundreds of people afflicted with cancer.

February 17th,1938 Arthur Connolly reports to Mr.Dupont on the latest action regarding the Connell patent application.
The Franklin Institute in a letter to Mr. Irenee Dupont dated 21st, February 1938 enclosed the agreement of termination of contract between the Hendry-Connell Research Foundation Limited and the Franklin Institute of the State of Pennsylvania for the Promotion of the Mechanic Arts, trustee of Biochemical Research Foundation,
This now places both foundations in the same position as they were before the original agreement was entered into.

Arthur Connelly still very keen on the research and clinical work going on in the Hendry-Connell Research Foundation. writes to Mr. Dupont enclosing a most interesting newspaper clipping from a Canadian paper. Also makes mention of the preparation of the third Bulletin and the antigenic properties found in Ensol.
Connolly is keeping Dupont fully informed of the activities at the Hendry-Connell Research Foundation in Kingston.

H.C.Connell continues to send to Dupont copies of typical letters received from physicians across the continent who report success using Ensol in their treatment of cancer. Also a number of them are forwarding needed tissue to the Kingston lab.

Also a number of these letters originating from outside of Canada contain interesting comparisons made between the two products "Rex" and "Ensol". There is one copy of a letter to Mr.Dupont from a Major M.J. Connolly thanking him for his financial part in producing the Ensol which was used in treating his wife Mrs. Connolly and so alleviated her pain when she was suffering so severely from terminal cancer. This note by coincidence is dated Sunday 3rd April 1938 the same day newspapers had headlines reporting the ten deaths in Orlando.

It is a surprise to the reviewer of this collection of Dupont papers that there really is no reference to the ten deaths that occurred in Orlando, Florida the last days of March and first days of April,1938. These deaths were found, after thorough investigation , to be caused by the contaminated product "Rex" shipped from Biochemical Research Foundation and used by Dr.T.A.Neal in treating his patients suffering from cancer. Dr. Neal had been using both products in his practice in Orlando, Ensol was cleared of any contamination by the Investigators. Dr. Neal continued to administer Ensol in his treatment to his patients suffering from cancer. and to report his results to Kingston.

Dr. Ellice Mcdonald director of the Biochemical Foundation in Philadelphia denied on Saturday 2nd April 1938, the possibility of any contamination occuring in the Philadelphia laboratory.

The lack of any letter from Mcdonald reporting to Dupont or any collection of newspaper clippings regarding the Orlando deaths in this file seems very much out of character.

It was a great misfortune that Ensol was ever mentioned as being the serum at fault.

The next piece is a copy of " the Journal of the American Medical Association " dated Saturday April 9th.1938 offering an opinion in the editorial that the Biochemical Research Foundation "prepared the product on a Friday and some of it was permitted to stand over Saturday and Sunday developing a toxin so that when sterilized on Monday an amount of tetanus toxin was present to cause death." If this was the case, the lack of a disciplined routine at the Philadelphia laboratory in preparing "Rex" reflected on "Ensol" with calamitous results.

In a letter of 12th April,'38 Mr. Dupont takes Dr. Stanley P. Reimann of the Lankenau Hospital in Philadelphia to task for his remark "maybe they should never have used Ensol in the beginning" reported in the papers. Dupont also encloses a copy of Bulletin No.3 of the Hendry-Connell Research Foundation. and also suggests that " researchers should stick together and encourage each other rather than the reverse". One wonders if that hospital enjoyed grants from Dupont sources !

15th April,38 Arthur Connolly writes to Dupont enclosing a very detailed letter

from Dr. Neal in Orlando to H.C.Connell in Kingston which gives an excellent
Dr. Neal's three page letter is most explicit and details most each hour of the
days in question. It is written by a brave and caring physician, setting out all
the relevant factors involved in this tragedy.
During the spring Dupont is forwarding the cause of Connell with the Federal
Government of Canada trying to get a license for the manufacture of Ensol.
Connell is trying to employ a full-time bacteriologist which is a governmental
requirement for the necessary license.

Irenee Dupont writes to H.C.Connell about his brother Pierre who has been
backing Dr. Kraemer for a number of years on his cancer work. showing the
family interest in finding a cancer remedy.

Dr.J.C.Connell(Hendry's father who was a director of the Foundation) writes
to Mr. Dupont regarding a tabulation of patients being prepared, **he also
mentions Dr. Neal, and writes, "your settlement with the unfortunate
families is a generous act indeed". This confirms the thinking of the
authors': that a cash settlement must have been made to the survivors but
never before confirmed !**

Dr.H.C. writes to Dupont 8th August'38 regarding a shipment of Ensol to
Dupont's friend Mr. Lipmann and that Dr.H.C. , Dr. Glen Burton and Dr. Neal
spoke together about Mr. Lipmann.
H.C. also spoke of the many difficulties he and Connolly were having with the
bureaucrats on the patent applications. this is a letter full of activities of
interest.

Another letter of 8th August'38 from Dr. J.C. to Dupont clarifying some
queries about patients records is probably Dupont's first real knowlege of how
Dr. Mundell behaved while director of the clinic in Kingston. Dr.J.C.. goes on
to explain that the opinions expressed by Dr. Mcdonald of the Kingston
operation would have all come from Mundell's sabotage.
There is a letter to Irenee from his brother Pierre (they both operated in the
same building) regarding Dr. Kraemar 's opinion of the Connell's last report
on treated patients. It would appear that the two brothers are certainly keenly
backing two different horses. One wonders if they are betting a few thousand
once in a while or did their father leave them the duty to find the cure for
cancer in their lifetime.

The late summer and fall of the year 1 9 3 8 brought a great deal of activity to
the Hendry-Connell Research Foundation and we will try to describe how it
moved along with reference to this correspondence..

A copy of a letter from Mitch Hepburn Premier of Ontario to Hendry Connell
advising that a commission was being set up to investigate cancer remedies and
to express through Hendry the government's appreciation to Mr. Irene Dupont

for his assistance to Hendry's outstanding work.

Further letters from patients and their doctors telling of successes in treatment using Ensol. Many telling of a reduction of pain but also reduction in size of tumors etc. **Newspaper clippings with a headline "Use of Ensol is approved in cancer therapy" dated Toronto November 15 (cp) 1938.**

There is a collection of letters regarding the health of Dupont's good friend Mr. Lippmann, who is suffering from cancer. Dr. Glenn Burton, director of the Kingston Clinic has travelled to Florida, New York and Cuba to visit and treat Mr. Lippmann. Burton has also met with Dr. Martinez and Dr.oOiode-Granda of the Cuban Cancer Institute through Mr. Dupont. Dr. Ellice Mcdonald was with Dupont in Cuba around November 16th/38. A letter from Dupont of November 25 to H.C.Connell congratulates and thanks him for sending a copy of a paper he had read at a meeting of the "Clinical Surgeons of Canada, Kingston, Ontario, Canada, October 7th, 1938". the paper was entitled " The Present Status of the Ensol Problem " and well received by those present.

The dates of the next lot of letters in the file run into the spring of 1939. At the end of April Mr. Dupont writes to Connolly telling him to call H.C.. Connell to tell him he cannot contribute $60,000.00 to keep the Institute going but will contribute $24,000.00 to give him a breathing space, pending a favourable action and decision by the Canadian Government. **He says he thinks "the outlook of convincing the Canadian Government is bright enough to warrant my gambling an additional $ 24,000.00 on behalf of the alleviation of human suffering."**

Mr. Connolly duly received 12 shares of Christiana Securities and reported to Mr. Dupont that he disposed of them at $ 2,030.00 per share for a net total of $24,239.40 and that he would deliver a cheque in that amount to Dr. Connell in Ottawa May 10th,1939 when they were to meet with certain members of the Dominion Government and also for the purpose of preparing an agreement whereby the Ontario Government will supervise the future progress of the Foundation.

It is interesting to note Connolly is still writing very enthusiastically and is most interested in all aspects of each effort. Of course he is still employed in the Legal Department, Patent Division of E.I.Dupont de Nemours & Company, Incorporated, Wilmington, Delaware.

so Mr. Irenee Dupont, whose office is in the same building must be approving of all his efforts on behalf of the Hendry-Connell Foundation.

There is a copy of the Annual Report of the President of the Hendry-Connell Research Foundation Limited for 1938-1939 reporting on the activities and progress with the two governments.

NOTE ----- It is from the date of the next letter -June 1st, 1939 --to the very last letter in this file -- April 23 rd 1946 -- roughly seven

years --that Dr Calvin Hendry Cameron Connell struggled, literally alone, to continue to produce and distribute "Ensol" for the relief from pain, and renewed hope of recovery of health for those patients being treated.
Some of these years of Hendry's lonely struggle are covered in chapters 8,9 and 10 of "Enzyme Solution --The Story of Ensol",
Therefore, the contents of some of these letters are a repeat of relevant details already reported, and will only be briefly noted.

H.C.Connell to Mr. Dupont 1st June 1938 reporting a resolution of the Board of Directors of the thanks due to Mr.Dupont from the board and from all those patients who have been given relief with new hope and comfort by the free distribution of Ensol. Also enclosed, a copy of the agreement between the Minister of Health of the Province of Ontario and the Foundation, completed and signed on 25th May 1939.

H.C.Connell writes 23rd November.1939 to Mr.Dupont asking for an interview and to have with him a representative of the Government of Ontario. He reports on the approval of Ensol by almost everyone but still the failure to secure a license from Department of Health Ottawa. Connell again requests continuation of " generous support"

Arthur Connolly writes to H.C.Connell 27th November 1939, advising Mr.Dupont sees no useful purpose in such a meeting or interview with government representative as proposed, **Dupont feels Ontario Government should take over production and distribution and that Federal Government should issue license because all available data warrants it. He speaks of the possiblity that some money might be available through CAPCO (see chapter 7 in publication) to assist in manufacture and distribution of Ensol for the next eight to ten month period with the expectation of obtaining the license from the Federal Government.**
Hendry writes to Dupont 11th December 1939 thanking him for his support and assuring Dupont of Hendry's every possible effort to justify the expenditures Dupont has made.

Dupont writes to Ellice Mcdonald 22nd May 1940 asking his opinion on a series of clinical histories from H.C.Connell. Mcdonald replies with a report from Dr. Murray Wright (who was **"struck with the length of time which many of these cases lived with fair comfort, because they did not receive any other treatment,their palliative results must be credited to Ensol."** no further comment by Mcdonald or Dupont,,,,,,.

This is a comment in a very interesting letter from Dupont to a Percy W. Philips dated 24 December, 1940 regarding charitable donations or contributions. It is not our intent or business to be any more concerned than how such contributions affected the Hendry-Connell Research Foundation . Mr. Dupont points out in the letter that since he became interested in cancer research he has contributed $1,784,657.54 the amount contributed to Hendry-Connell Research Foundation in Kingston is small indeed to the amounts contributed to other organizations "approved " as charitable organizations. He writes to the Internal Revenue Department that " it would be very disasteful to me to face the likelihood of having to pay a large gift tax on such contribution as I may make, and I should like a very prompt withdrawal of this claim of the Internal Revenue department that such a gift is taxable".

H.C.Connell writes to Dupont on 6th September 1941 about having received a questionnaire form from the US Teasury dept. regarding the Foundation which he promptly completed and returned. **Connell also reports that the Ontario Cancer Commission reports that Ensol is now recommended as a remedy which can be used without harm and that it gives beneficial results in a large percentage of cases.**

There is a letter to Mr. Dupont from Dr. Allen J. Fleming of the Haskell Laboratory of Industrial Toxicology in Wilmington Delaware thanking him for information on the tax situation with respect to aiding cancer research in Canada.

Arthur Conolly writes to Hendry Connell on 2nd April ,1942 that the Court of Appeals has reversed the District Court and as a result held that Ensol was a patentable invention. In view of this , Connolly advises Hendry of a number of steps he should take to ensure that the patent is properly negotiable and available when required by a manufacturing firm.

H.C.Connell writes to Mr. Dupont 18th March,1942 of the clinical results improving and the Ontario Government giving $3,000.00 a month, barely enough to meet all obligations. Ensol still being shipped free Also Hendry has renounced all personal interest in Ensol patents. He asks Mr. Dupont if he can consent to the reassignment of the Canadian patent to the Ontario Government.. **This move would refute the statements and innuendoes circulating that Connell is exploiting Ensol for his own personal advantage.**

H.C.Connell replies to Mr, Dupont on 6th July,1942 regarding his letter concerning a friend of his brother Lammot. Hendry offers to care personally for this person if his condition warrants the long trip to Kingston. Hendry takes this opportunity to report on activities and also offers to forward for Mr. Dupont's viewing a copy of a colour film with sound entitled **'A Serological Approach to the Treatment of Malignant Disease'**. This was produced by Professor Munro of Queen's University, Donald Alexander and Hendry. **The Cancer Commission, after viewing it had favourable comments although they were of the opinion that**

14

indiscriminate showing would result in a rush of patients. Hendry states the film is scientific and not intended for the laity.

The film has also been shown to two or three medical societies and their reactions were all one could desire. Hendry states it would be well to wait until they can put a more potent antigen than that now present before making further attempts to license Ensol.

(This film has not yet been recovered)

There are two letters dated 1st and 3rd October 1942 referring to receipts covering Mr Duponts payment to Price Waterhouse for their review of Hendry-Connell Research Foundation books over a five year period.

Arthur Connolly writes to Mr. Dupont with the news that Connell's US patent on Ensol has finally been issued and encloses a copy. This success is the result of seven years fighting with various tribunals involved. Mr.Dupont replies 20th April with his congratulations and states he wants to be kept posted on any developments that may occur.

An interesting note-- December 13th, 1946 a letter from Irenee Dupont to Dr. Ellice Mcdonald states Dupont's reasoning for refusing to recommend contributing a centrifuge to the Biochemical lab.

==

13th February, 1946 Arthur G Connolly writes to Irenee Dupont that he is happy to advise that the Canadian Government has finally granted the Hendry-Connell Research Foundation, Limited a license (no.93) to manufacture and sell the cancer serum of the Connell patent throughout the Dominion of Canada.

23rd April, 1946 Irenee Dupont replies to Connolly, on his return from Cuba congratulating him and the doctors Connell on finally getting this permit.

==

Epilogue

It is regrettable that the work of The Hendry-Connell Research Foundation was neither completely understood nor fully appreciated in Canada by those contemporaries in charge of the development and financing of such endeavours. It is impossible to guess what might have been achieved had the active support promised, been forthcoming at that time.

On May 21, 2001 an interesting report appeared in the TORONTO GLOBE AND MAIL: The Federal Government is investing $60 Million in a ten year program by the Canadian arm of the French drug giant AVENTIS to develop a cancer vaccine nearly six decades after Calvin Hendry Cameron Connell first produced an antigen which was first thought to be an enzyme which he named ENSOL. (left in his papers for safekeeping is a procedure for a cancer vaccine) Queen's University Archives, Kingston, Ontario, Canada, protects The Hendry-Connell Research Foundation papers.

It is to be hoped this book will encourage some researcher somewhere sometime to further develop Dr. Connell's thirty-year research and prove the prediction he made before he died in 1964,

"it is from this particular field,
namely the study of the serological processes
involved in immunity and disease,
that, success in treatment and control of cancer
will be found."

Hendry C. Connell 1895-1964

16

KINGSTON LABORATORY

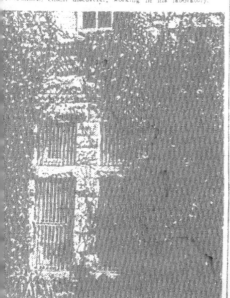

C Cohnell, ensoll discoverer, working in his laboratory.

Sanctions Issue Splits Laborites; Leader May Quit

Willing to Ride Rods to Prison

La Crosse, Wis., Oct. 1.—(UP)
When John Bodak, 21, surrendered to police to-day and told them he was an escaped convict from a Mansfield, O., prison, authorities wired Mansfield and offered to return the man. But Mansfield replied there was no money. "O.K.," said Bodak, "I'll ride the rods back; it looks like a long, cold Winter ahead."

Squirrel Season Set for Hunters

Regulations Changed in Numerous Respects, Nixon Announces.

ADVANCE DEER SEASON

Two days open season for black and grey squirrels—Thursday, Oct. 24, and Friday, Oct. 25—in that section of Ontario lying south of the French and Mattawa rivers, has been authorized by order-in-Council of the Hepburn Government, it was announced yesterday by Hon. Harry C. Nixon, minister of game and fisheries.

Hunters will be limited to a bag of five squirrels per day. All squirrels taken must either be used for food or mounted as trophies.

The squirrel season—the first general season for this type of game in many years—was only one of a number of hunting regulation changes announced by Mr. Nixon. Others include an open deer season in Carleton County, from Nov. 5 to Nov. 20; a moose season for Renfrew County, Nov. 5 to Nov. 20; a wild goose season for Kent and Essex Counties, from Oct. 15 to Dec. 14; an otter season from Nov. 1, 1935 to Feb. 28, 1936; and two days pheasant shooting on Pelee Island, Oct. 23 and Oct. 24.

The Government has also advanced the deer season by four days in the Rainy River district and that part of Kenora and Thunder Bay lying south of the Canadian National Railway. Originally this season was to start on Oct. 21. It now will commence on Oct. 25.

The Pelee Island pheasant shooting precedes by two days elaborate field trials for dogs on the island. The birds are reportedly very plentiful. The township of Pelee has been au-

Pacifist Lansbury Believes Force Gets Nobody Anything.

PARTY CONVENTION

Vote Expected To-day Following Bitter Controversy.

Brighton, England, Oct. 1.—(AP)—The question of sanctions against Premier Mussolini in the event of an Italo-Ethiopian war to-day led to violent controversy between party leaders in the first session of the Labor party convention.

A bitter debate was climaxed by George Lansbury's re-affirmation of his offer to quit as the party leader in the House of Commons. He called his position "intolerable."

Although the vote to be taken tomorrow is expected to show the party overwhelmingly in favor of using sanctions against Italy if necessary, Lansbury may not be required to quit, despite his expressed pacifist convictions.

That was indicated by the manner in which the convention suddenly united in a spectacular personal tribute to the party leader.

Lansbury himself hinted that he might continue as leader, declaring that the subject of the sanctions debate "is not the overwhelming, fundamental question that brings us together."

Bitter and Difficult

"I want every one to understand," said Lansbury, "that it is bitter and difficult for me to stand here and publicly repudiate this big fundamental policy (for sanctions). I agree it is quite intolerable that you should have a man speaking as a leader who disagrees fundamentally with issues of this kind.

"I have had to speak for the party, and I have had to see Sir Samuel Hoare for the party, but on each occasion I have tried honestly, and straightforwardly to state the party position."

He said the Labor members of parliament will decide his fate next week because "this conference obviously is unable to deal with the matter except by some kind of an emergency motion making recommendation to the parliamentary party."

Lansbury's personal stand against sanctions was born of his belief that "force never can, never has and never will bring permanent peace and good will to the world."

Sir Stafford Cripps, left wing Laborite, assailed the sanctions policy and was attacked for his stand by late speakers.

Ernest Bevin accused Cripps of "doing his best to split the party." Joh

Made in the USA